11/28/22

3rd edition
High-Yield Neuroanatomy

3rd edition
High-Yield Neuroanatomy

James D. Fix, Ph.D.

Professor Emeritus of Anatomy

Marshall University School of Medicine

Huntington, West Virginia

LIPPINCOTT WILLIAMS & WILKINS

A **Wolters Kluwer** Company

Philadelphia · Baltimore · New York · London
Buenos Aires · Hong Kong · Sydney · Tokyo

Acquisitions Editors: Betty Sun
Development Editor: Louise Bierig
Managing Editor: Scott Scheidt
Marketing Manager: Joe Schott
Production Editor: Sirkka E. H. Bertling
Designer: Holly McLaughlin
Compositor: Maryland Composition
Printer: Data Reproductions Corporation

351 West Camden Street
Baltimore, MD 21201

530 Walnut Street
Philadelphia, PA 19106

Printed in the United States of America

First Edition, 1995
Second Edition, 2000

Library of Congress Cataloging-in-Publication Data

Fix, James D.
　　High-yield neuroanatomy / James D. Fix. — 3rd ed.
　　　　　p. ; cm.
　　Includes bibliographical references and index.
　　ISBN 13: 978-0-7817-5899-4
　　ISBN 10: 0-7817-5899-8
　　1. Neuroanatomy—Outlines, syllabi, etc. 2. Neuroanatomy—Examination, questions, etc. I. Title.
　　[DNLM: 1. Nervous System—anatomy & histology—Examination Questions. 2. Nervous System—anatomy & histology—Outlines. 3. Nervous System Diseases—Examination Questions. 4. Nervous System Diseases—Outlines. WL 18.2 F566h 2005]
　　QM451.F588 2005
　　611.8'076—dc22

　　　　　　　　　　　　　　　　　　　　　　　　　　　　　　2004061558

The publishers have made every effort to trace the copyright holders for borrowed material. If they have inadvertently overlooked any, they will be pleased to make the necessary arrangements at the first opportunity.

To purchase additional copies of this book, call our customer service department at **(800) 638-3030** or fax orders to **(301) 824-7390**. International customers should call **(301) 714-2324**.

Visit Lippincott Williams & Wilkins on the Internet: http://www.LWW.com. Lippincott Williams & Wilkins customer service representatives are available from 8:30 am to 6:00 pm, EST.

　　　　　　　　　　　　　　　　　　　　　　　　　　　　　　　　　　　　08
　　　　　　　　　　　　　　　　　　　　　　　　3 4 5 6 7 8 9 10

Preface

....

The third edition of *High-Yield Neuroanatomy* is still neuroanatomy at its irreducible minimum, containing most, if not all, of the national board themes. The sole purpose of the book is to get you through the nervous system topics covered on the United States Medical Licensing Examination (USMLE) Step 1. Substantial additions have been made to accommodate student requests and suggestions.

NEW TO THIS EDITION
- Neurohistology Case Studies
- Mini-atlas of nuclear magnetic imaging scans
- Carotid and vertebral digital subtraction angiography
- Nuclear magnetic angiography
- Additional figures of cross-sectional anatomy of the brain

TO THE STUDENT
To make the most of this book, study the illustrations, computed tomography scans, and magnetic resonance images carefully, and read the legends. Many board-type questions come from this source. In fact, the answers to at least 20 common USMLE questions are found within this preface. Finally, remember these tips as you scan the chapters:

Chapter 1: The mini-atlas provides you with the essential examination structures labeled on computed tomography scans and magnetic resonance images.

Chapter 2: Cerebrospinal fluid pathways are well demonstrated in Figure 2-1. Cerebrospinal fluid is produced by the choroid plexus and absorbed by the arachnoid villi that jut into the venous sinuses.

Chapter 3: The essential arteries and the functional areas that they irrigate are shown. Study the carotid and vertebral angiograms and the epidural and subdural hematomas in computed tomography scans and magnetic resonance images.

Chapter 4: The neural crest and its derivatives, the dual origin of the pituitary gland, and the difference between spina bifida and the Arnold-Chiari malformation are presented. Study the figures that illustrate the Arnold-Chiari and Dandy-Walker malformations.

Chapter 5: What is the difference between Lewy and Hirano bodies? Nerve cells contain Nissl substance in their perikarya and dendrites, but not in their axons. Remember that Nissl substance (rough endoplasmic reticulum) plays a role in protein synthesis. Study Figure 5-3 on the localization and prevalence of common brain and spinal cord tumors. Remember that, in adults, glioblastoma multiforme is the most common brain tumor, followed by astrocytoma and meningioma. In children, astrocytoma is the most common brain tumor, followed by medulloblastoma and ependymoma. In the spinal cord, ependymoma is the most common tumor.

Chapter 6: The adult spinal cord terminates (conus terminalis) at the lower border of the first lumbar vertebra. The newborn's spinal cord extends to the third lumbar vertebra. In adults, the cauda equina extends from vertebral levels L-2 to Co.

Chapter 7: The tracts of the spinal cord are reduced to four: corticospinal (pyramidal), dorsal columns, pain and temperature, and Horner's. Know them cold.

Chapter 8: Study the eight classic national board lesions of the spinal cord. Four heavy hitters are: Brown-Siquard syndrome, B_{12} avitaminosis (subacute combined degeneration), syringomyelia, and amyotrophic lateral sclerosis (Lou Gehrig's disease).

Chapter 9: Study the transverse sections of the brain stem, and localize the cranial nerve nuclei. Study the ventral surface of the brain stem, and identify the exiting and entering cranial nerves. On the dorsal surface of the brain stem, identify the only exiting cranial nerve, the trochlear nerve.

Chapter 10: Cranial nerve (CN) V-1 is the afferent limb of the corneal reflex. CN V-1, CN V-2, CN III, CN IV, CN VI, and the postganglionic sympathetic fibers are all found in the cavernous sinus.

Chapter 11: Figure 11-1 shows the auditory pathway. What are the causes of conduction and sensorineural deafness? Describe the Weber and Rinne tuning fork tests. Remember that the auditory nerve and the organ of Corti are derived from the otic placode.

Chapter 12: This chapter describes the two types of vestibular nystagmus: postrotational and caloric (COWS acronym). Vestibulo-ocular reflexes in the unconscious patient are also discussed (see Figure 12-3).

Chapter 13: This chapter on the cranial nerves is pivotal. It spawns more neuroanatomy examination questions than any other chapter. Carefully study all of the figures and legends. The seventh cranial nerve deserves special consideration (see Figures 13-5 and 13-6). Understand the difference between an upper motor neuron and a lower motor neuron (Bell's palsy).

Chapter 14: The three most important lesions of the brain stem are occlusion of the anterior spinal artery (Figure 14-1), occlusion of the posterior inferior cerebellar artery (Figure 14-1), and medial longitudinal fasciculus syndrome (Figure 14-2). Weber's syndrome is the most common midbrain lesion (Figure 14-3).

Chapter 15: Figure 15-1 shows the most important cerebellar circuit. The inhibitory γ-aminobutyric acid (GABA)-ergic Purkinje cells give rise to the cerebellodentatothalamic tract. What are mossy and climbing fibers?

Chapter 16: Figure 16-1 shows everything you need to know about what goes in and what comes out of the thalamus. Know the anatomy of the internal capsule; it will be on the examination. What is the blood supply of the internal capsule (stroke)?

Chapter 17: Know the lesions of the visual system. How are quadrantanopias created? There are two major lesions of the optic chiasma. Know them! What is Meyer's loop?

Chapter 18: The important anatomy of the autonomic nervous system is clearly seen in Figures 18-1 and 18-2.

Chapter 19: Figures 19-1 and 19-2 show that the paraventricular and supraoptic nuclei synthesize and release antidiuretic hormone and oxytocin. The suprachiasmatic nucleus receives direct input from the retina and plays a role in the regulation of circadian rhythms.

Chapter 20: Bilateral lesions of the amygdala result in Klüver-Bucy syndrome. Recall the triad hyperphagia, hypersexuality, and psychic blindness. Memory loss is associated with bilateral lesions of the hippocampus. Wernicke's encephalopathy results from a deficiency of thiamine (vitamin B_1). Lesions are found in the mamillary bodies, thalamus, and midbrain tegmentum (Figure 20-3). Know the Papez circuit, a common board question.

Chapter 21: Figure 21-6 shows the circuitry of the basal ganglia and their associated neurotransmitters. Parkinson's disease is associated with a depopulation of neurons in the substantia nigra. Huntington's disease results in a loss of nerve cells in the caudate nucleus and putamen. Hemiballism results from infarction of the contralateral subthalamic nucleus.

Chapter 22: In this chapter, the pathways of the major neurotransmitters are shown in separate brain maps. Glutamate is the major excitatory transmitter of the brain; GABA is the major inhibitory transmitter. Purkinje cells of the cerebellum are GABA-ergic. In Alzheimer's disease, there is a loss of acetylcholinergic neurons in the basal nucleus of Meynert. In Parkinson's disease, there is a loss of dopaminergic neurons in the substantia nigra.

Chapter 23: This chapter describes the cortical localization of functional areas of the brain. How does the dominant hemisphere differ from the nondominant hemisphere? Figure 23-5 shows the effects of various major hemispheric lesions. What symptoms result from a lesion of the right inferior parietal lobe? What is Gerstmann's syndrome?

Chapter 24: This chapter describes apraxia, aphasia, and dysprosody. Be able to differentiate Broca's aphasia from Wernicke's aphasia. What is conduction aphasia? This is board-relevant material.

I wish you good luck.

James D. Fix

Acknowledgments

···

I wish to thank my medical students, colleagues, and members of the staff of Lippincott Williams & Wilkins for their valuable comments, suggestions, and help. Thanks also go to Louise Bierig for her editorial direction.

Contents

···

1

Cross-Sectional Anatomy of the Brain

I. INTRODUCTION. The illustrations in this chapter are accompanied by corresponding magnetic resonance imaging (MRI) scans. Together they represent a **mini-atlas** of brain slices in the three orthogonal planes (i.e., midsagittal, coronal, and axial). An insert on each figure shows the level of the slice. The most commonly tested structures are labeled.

II. MIDSAGITTAL SECTION. (Figures 1-1, 1-2, and 1-3). The location of the structures shown in the figures should be known.

III. CORONAL SECTION THROUGH THE OPTIC CHIASM (Figures 1-4 and 1-5). The location of the structures shown in the figures should be known.

Figure 1-1. Midsagittal section of the brain and brain stem showing the structures surrounding the third and fourth ventricles. The brain stem includes the midbrain (M), pons (P), and medulla oblongata.

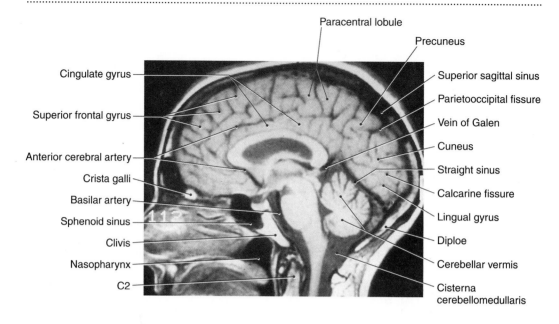

Figure 1-2. Midsagittal magnetic resonance imaging section through the brain and brain stem showing the important structures surrounding the third and fourth ventricles. This is a T1-weighted image. The gray matter is gray (hypointense), whereas the white matter is white (hyperintense).

Figure 1-3. Midsagittal magnetic resonance imaging section through the brain stem and diencephalon. Note the cerebrospinal fluid tract: lateral ventricle, interventricular foramen of Monro, third ventricle, cerebral aqueduct, fourth ventricle, foramen of Magendie, cerebellomedullary cistern, and spinal subarachnoid space. Note also the relation between the optic chiasm, infundibulum, and hypophysis (pituitary gland).

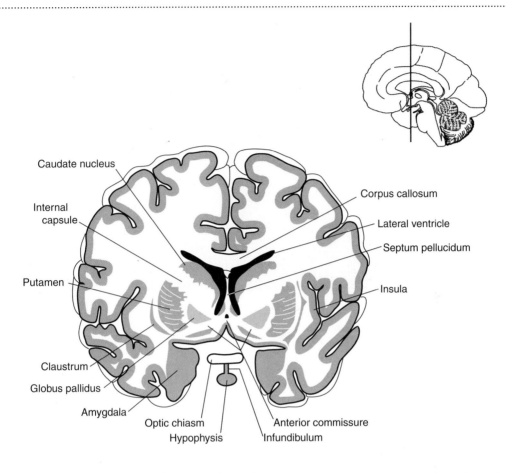

Figure 1-4. Coronal section of the brain at the level of the anterior commissure, optic chiasm, and amygdala. Note that the internal capsule lies between the caudate nucleus and the lentiform nucleus (globus pallidus and putamen).

IV. CORONAL SECTION THROUGH THE MAMILLARY BODIES (Figures 1-6 and 1-7). The location of the structures shown in the figures should be known.

V. AXIAL IMAGE THROUGH THE THALAMUS AND INTERNAL CAPSULE (Figures 1-8 and 1-9). The location of the structures shown in the figures should be known.

VI. AXIAL IMAGE THROUGH THE MIDBRAIN, MAMILLARY BODIES, AND OPTIC TRACT (Figures 1-10, 1-11, 1-12, and 1-13). The location of the structures shown in the figures should be known.

VII. ATLAS OF THE BRAIN AND BRAIN STEM (FIGURES 1-14–1-24) Includes mid-sagittal, parasagittal, coronal and axial sections of thick stained brain slices.

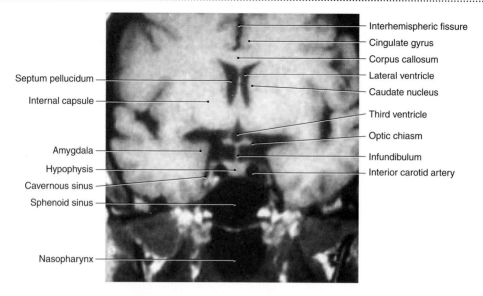

Septum pellucidum
Internal capsule

Amygdala
Hypophysis
Cavernous sinus
Sphenoid sinus

Nasopharynx

Interhemispheric fissure
Cingulate gyrus
Corpus callosum
Lateral ventricle
Caudate nucleus
Third ventricle
Optic chiasm
Infundibulum
Interior carotid artery

Figure 1-5.   Coronal magnetic resonance imaging section through the amygdala, optic chiasma, infundibulum, and internal capsule. The cavernous sinus encircles the sella turcica and contains the following structures: cranial nerves (CN) III, IV, VI, V-1, and V-2; postganglionic sympathetic fibers; and the internal carotid artery. This is a T1-weighted image.

Lateral ventricle
Fornix
Internal capsule
Corpus callosum
Caudate nucleus
Third ventricle
Thalamus
Insula
Putamen
Globus pallidus
Lateral ventricle
Subthalamic nucleus
Substantia nigra
Mamillary bodies
Infundibulum
Optic tract
Hippocampus

Figure 1-6.   Coronal section of the brain at the level of the thalamus, mamillary bodies, and hippocampal formation. Note that the internal capsule lies between the thalamus and the lentiform nucleus.

Figure 1-7. Coronal magnetic resonance imaging section of the brain and brain stem at the level of the thalamus, and hippocampal formation. Note that the posterior limb of the internal capsule lies between the thalamus and the lentiform nucleus (putamen and globus pallidus). This is a T1-weighted postcontrast image.

Figure 1-8. Axial section of the brain at the level of the internal capsule and basal ganglia. Note that the internal capsule has an anterior limb, a genu, and a posterior limb. Note also that the corpus callosum is sectioned through the genu and splenium.

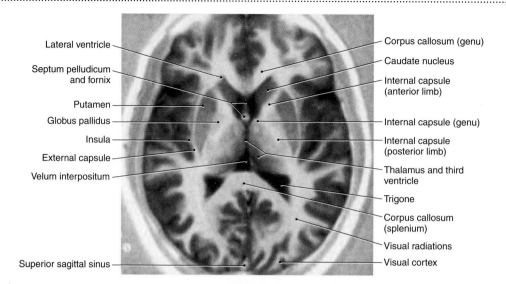

Lateral ventricle

Septum pelludicum and fornix

Putamen

Globus pallidus

Insula

External capsule

Velum interpositum

Superior sagittal sinus

Corpus callosum (genu)

Caudate nucleus

Internal capsule (anterior limb)

Internal capsule (genu)

Internal capsule (posterior limb)

Thalamus and third ventricle

Trigone

Corpus callosum (splenium)

Visual radiations

Visual cortex

Figure 1-9.   Axial magnetic resonance imaging section at the level of the internal capsule and basal ganglia. Note that the caudate nucleus bulges into the frontal horn of the lateral ventricle. In Huntington's disease, there is a massive loss of γ-aminobutyric acid (GABA)-ergic neurons in the caudate nucleus that results in hydrocephalus ex vacuo. A lesion of the genu of the internal capsule results in a contralateral weak lower face with sparing of the upper face. This is a T1-weighted image.

Optic tract

Basis pedunculi

Lateral ventricle

Third ventricle

Mamillary body

Amygdala

CN III

Substantia nigra

Red nucleus

Hippocampus

Trochlear nucleus

Nucleus of inferior colliculus

Cerebral aqueduct

Cerebellum

Figure 1-10.   Axial section of the brain at the level of the midbrain, mamillary bodies, and amygdala. Note that the substantia nigra separates the crus cerebri from the tegmentum of the midbrain.

Interhemispheric fissure

Gyrus rectus

Optic tract

Mamillary nucleus

Red nucleus

Trigone

Superior colliculus

Middle cerebral artery

Uncus / amygdala

Crus cerebri

Substantia nigra

Posterior cerebral artery

Quadrigeminal cistern

Cerebellar vermis

Straight sinus

Superior sagittal sinus

Figure 1-11.   Axial magnetic resonance imaging (MRI) section at the level of the midbrain and mamillary bodies. Because of the high iron content, the red nuclei, mamillary bodies, and substantia nigri show a reduced MRI signal in T2-weighted images. Flowing blood in the cerebral vessels stands out as a signal void. Cerebrospinal fluid produces a strong signal in the ventricles and cisterns.

Optic nerve

Optic nerve

Amygdala

Optic chiasm

Optic tract

Infundibulum

Mamillary bodies

Crus cerebri

Substantia nigra

Cerebral aqueduct

Lateral ventricle
(temporal horn)

Cerebellar vermis

Lateral ventricle
(occipital horn)

Superior sagittal sinus

Figure 1-12.   Axial magnetic resonance imaging section at the level of the optic chiasm, mamillary bodies, and midbrain. This patient has neurofibromatis type 1 and an optic nerve glioma. Note the size of the right optic nerve. The infundibulum is postfixed. This is a T1-weighted image.

Figure 1–13. Axial magnetic resonance imaging section at the level of the uncal incisure, oculomotor nerve, and inferior colliculus. Is there pathology within the orbit?

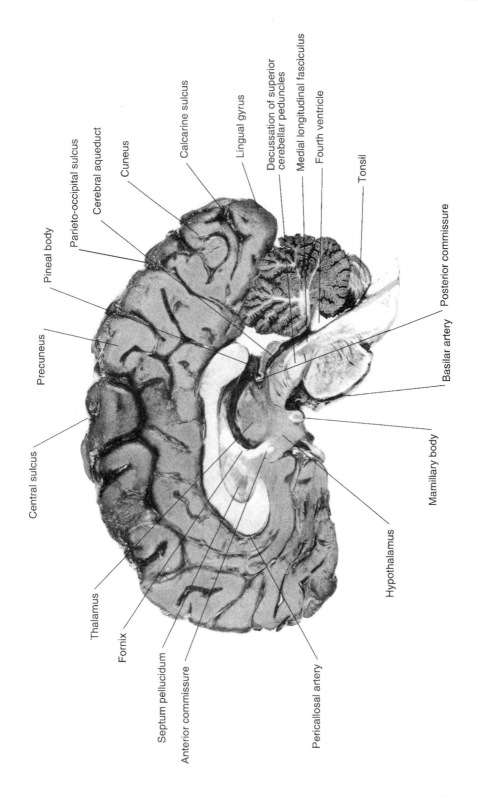

Figure 1–14. Gross midsagittal section of the brain and brain stem with meninges and blood vessels intact. Arachnoid granulations are seen along the crest of the hemisphere. The posterior commissure, decussation of the superior cerebellar peduncles, and medial longitudinal fasciculus are well demonstrated. (Reprinted with permission from Roberts M, Hanaway J, Morest DK: *Atlas of the Human Brain in Section*, 2nd ed. Philadelphia, Lea & Febiger, 1987, p. 85.)

Figure 1–15.   Gross parasagittal section through the red nucleus, medial lemniscus, and inferior olivary nucleus. The corticospinal fibers can be traced from the crus cerebri to the spinal cord. The abducent nerve (CN VI) is seen exiting from the pontobullar sulcus. (Reprinted with permission from Roberts M, Hanaway J, Morest DK: *Atlas of the Human Brain in Section*, 2nd ed. Philadelphia, Lea & Febiger, 1987, p. 81.)

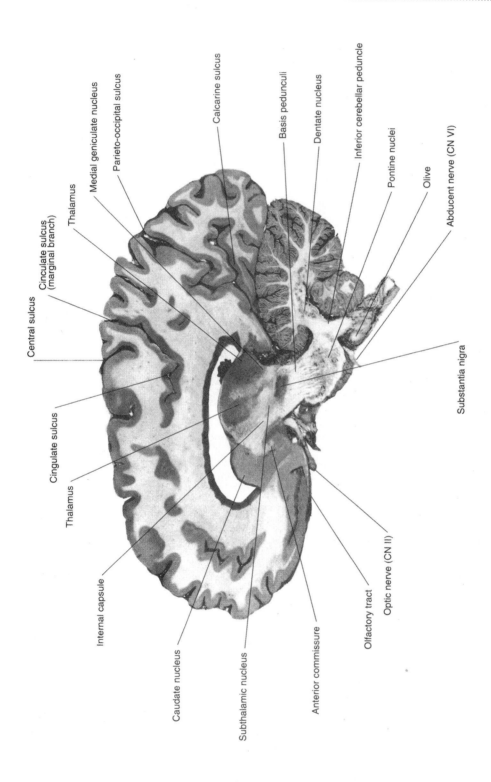

Figure 1–16. Gross parasagittal section through the caudate nucleus, subthalamic nucleus, substantia nigra, and dentate nucleus. The abducent nerve (CN VI) is seen exiting the pontobulbar sulcus. Damage to the subthalamic nucleus results in hemiballism. Parkinson disease results from a cell loss of the pigmented neurons in the substantia nigra. (Reprinted with permission from Roberts M, Hanaway J, Morest DK: *Atlas of the Human Brain in Section*, 2nd ed. Philadelphia, Lea & Febiger, 1987, p. 79.)

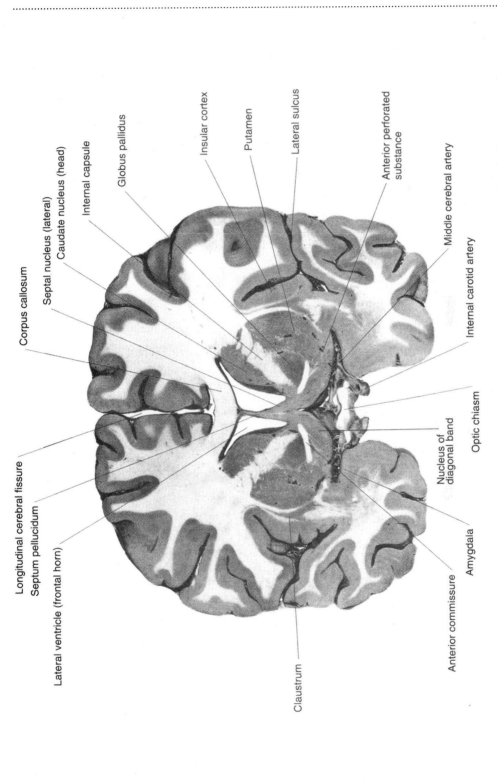

Longitudinal cerebral fissure
Septum pellucidum
Lateral ventricle (frontal horn)
Corpus callosum
Septal nucleus (lateral)
Caudate nucleus (head)
Internal capsule
Globus pallidus
Insular cortex
Putamen
Lateral sulcus
Anterior perforated substance
Middle cerebral artery
Internal carotid artery
Optic chiasm
Nucleus of diagonal band
Amygdala
Anterior commissure
Claustrum

Figure 1–17. Coronal section through the anterior commissure, amygdala, septal nuclei, and optic chiasm. The septal nuclei have reciprocal connections with the hippocampal formation (subiculum). (Reprinted with permission from Roberts M, Hanaway J, Morest DK: *Atlas of the Human Brain in Section*, 2nd ed. Philadelphia, Lea & Febiger, 1987, p. 9.)

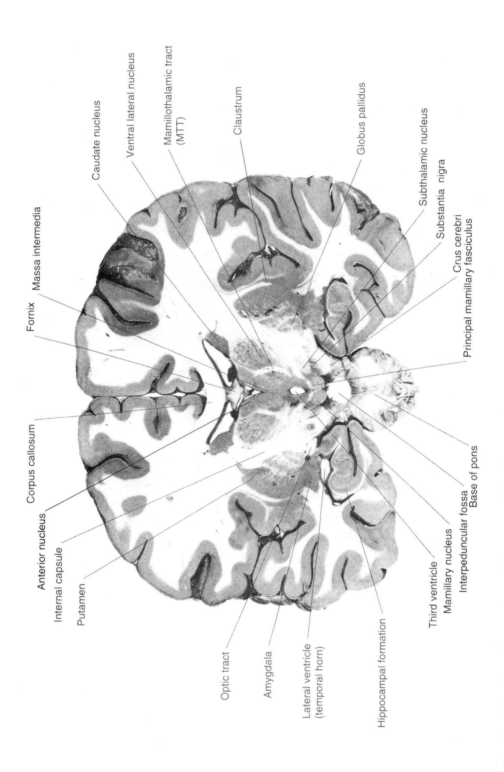

Figure 1–18. Coronal section through the posterior limb of the internal capsule, mamillothalamic tract (*MTT*), mamillary body, and hippocampal formation. Note the MTT entering the anterior ventral nucleus. The optic tracts are visible bilaterally. (Reprinted with permission from Roberts M, Hanaway J, Morest DK: *Atlas of the Human Brain in Section*, 2nd ed. Philadelphia, Lea & Febiger, 1987, p. 19.)

Caudate nucleus

Ventral lateral nucleus

Mamillothalamic tract (MTT)

Claustrum

Globus pallidus

Subthalamic nucleus

Substantia nigra

Crus cerebri

Principal mamillary fasciculus

Massa intermedia

Fornix

Corpus callosum

Anterior nucleus

Internal capsule

Putamen

Optic tract

Amygdala

Lateral ventricle (temporal horn)

Hippocampal formation

Third ventricle

Mamillary nucleus

Interpeduncular fossa

Base of pons

Figure 1–19. Coronal section through the thalamus, ventral posteromedial nucleus (*VPM*) and the ventral posterolateral nucleus (*VPL*), posterior limb of the internal capsule, substantia nigra, and red nucleus. The optic tract lies dorsal to the temporal horn of the lateral ventricle. (Reprinted with permission from Roberts M, Hanaway J, Morest DK: *Atlas of the Human Brain in Section,* 2nd ed. Philadelphia, Lea & Febiger, 1987, p. 23.)

Figure 1–20.   Coronal section through the lateral and medial lemnisci, lateral and medial geniculate nuclei, and hippocampal formation. (Reprinted with permission from Roberts M, Hanaway J, Morest DK: *Atlas of the Human Brain in Section*, 2nd ed. Philadelphia, Lea & Febiger, 1987, p. 25.)

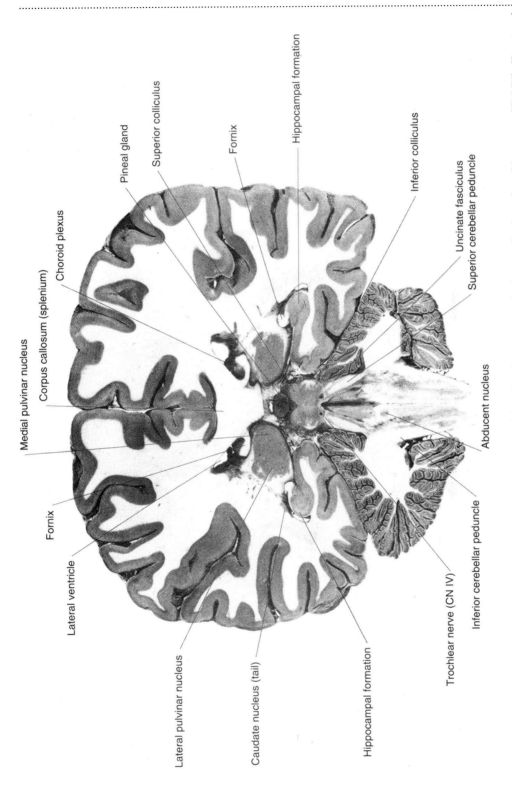

Figure 1–21.   Coronal section through the pulvinar nuclei, pineal gland (epiphysis), superior and inferior colliculi, and trochlear nerve (CN IV). (Reprinted with permission from Roberts M, Hanaway J, Morest DK: *Atlas of the Human Brain in Section*, 2nd ed. Philadelphia, Lea & Febiger, 1987, p. 29.)

Figure 1–22. Axial section through the internal capsule, anterior commissure, and pulvinar nuclei. (Reprinted with permission from Roberts M, Hanaway J, Morest DK: *Atlas of the Human Brain in Section*, 2nd ed. Philadelphia, Lea & Febiger, 1987, p. 51.)

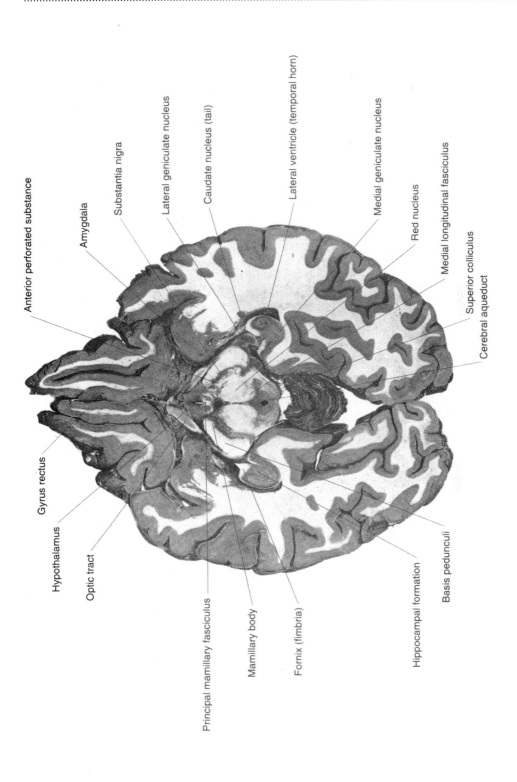

Figure 1–23. Axial section through the mamillary nuclei and the superior colliculi. (Reprinted with permission from Roberts M, Hanaway J, Morest DK: *Atlas of the Human Brain in Section*, 2nd ed. Philadelphia, Lea & Febiger, 1987, p. 57.)

Figure 1–24. Axial section through the mamillary nuclei, optic chiasm, and inferior colliculi. (Reprinted with permission from Roberts M, Hanaway J, Morest DK: *Atlas of the Human Brain in Section*, 2nd ed. Philadelphia, Lea & Febiger, 1987, p. 59.)

Labels on figure:

- Medial longitudinal fasciculus
- Parahippocampal gyrus
- Lateral lemniscus
- Substantia nigra
- Basis pedunculi
- Cerebral aqueduct
- Optic tract
- Cerebellum
- Olfactory tract
- Inferior colliculus
- Gyrus rectus
- Optic chiasm
- Amygdala
- Anterior commissure
- Lateral ventricle (temporal horn)
- Mamillary body
- Hippocampal formation
- Dentothalamic tract (Sup. cerebellar peduncle)

2

Meninges, Ventricles, and Cerebrospinal Fluid

I. MENINGES are three **connective tissue membranes** that surround the spinal cord and brain.

A. They consist of the **pia mater, arachnoid,** and **dura mater.**

1. The **pia mater** is a delicate, highly vascular layer of connective tissue. It closely covers the surface of the brain and spinal cord.

2. The **arachnoid** is a delicate, nonvascular connective tissue membrane. It is located between the dura mater and the pia mater.

3. The **dura mater** is the outer layer of meninges. It consists of dense connective tissue.

B. Meningial spaces

1. The **subarachnoid space** (Figure 2-1) lies between the pia mater and the arachnoid. It terminates at the level of the second sacral vertebra. It contains the cerebrospinal fluid (CSF).

2. Subdural space

a. In the **cranium,** the subdural space is traversed by "bridging" veins.

b. In the **spinal cord,** it is a clinically insignificant potential space.

3. Epidural space

a. The **cranial epidural space** is a potential space. It contains the meningeal arteries and veins.

b. The **spinal epidural space** contains fatty areolar tissue, lymphatics, and venous plexuses. The epidural space may be injected with a local anesthetic to produce a paravertebral ("saddle") nerve block.

C. Meningial tumors

1. **Meningiomas** are benign, well-circumscribed, slow-growing tumors. They account for 15% of primary intracranial tumors and are more common in women than in men (3:2). Ninety percent of meningiomas are supratentorial.

2. Subdural and epidural hematomas

a. **Subdural hematoma** is caused by laceration of the superior cerebral (bridging) veins.

b. **Epidural hematoma** is caused by laceration of the middle meningeal artery.

Figure 2-1. The subarachnoid spaces and cisterns of the brain and spinal cord. Cerebrospinal fluid is produced in the choroid plexuses of the ventricles. It exits the fourth ventricle, circulates in the subarachnoid space, and enters the superior sagittal sinus through the arachnoid granulations. Note that the conus medullaris terminates at L-1. The lumbar cistern ends at S-2. (Reprinted with permission from Noback CR, Strominger NL, Demarest R: *The Human Nervous System*, 4th ed. Baltimore, Williams & Wilkins, 1991, p. 68.)

D. Trauma

E. Meningitis is inflammation of the pia–arachnoid area of the brain, the spinal cord, or both.

    1. Bacterial meningitis is characterized clinically by fever, headache, nuchal rigidity, and Kernig's sign. (With the patient supine, the examiner flexes the patient's hip but cannot extend the knee without causing pain. It is a sign of meningeal irritation.) [**Remember: Kernig = knee.**] More than 70% of cases occur in children younger than 5 years of age. The disease may cause cranial nerve palsies and hydrocephalus.

a. Common causes

(1) in newborns (<1 month), bacterial meningitis is most frequently caused by *Group B streptococci (Streptococcus agalactiae), E. coli, and Listeria monocytogenes*

(2) in older infants and young children (1–23 months), it is most commonly caused by *Streptococcus pneumoniae.*

(3) in young adults (2–18 years), it is most frequently caused by *Neisseria meningitidis.*

(4) In older adults (19 years and older), it is most frequently caused by *Streptococcus pneumoniae.*
NB: Immunization against Hemophilis influenzae has significantly reduced this type of meningitis.

b. CSF findings

(1) Numerous polymorphonuclear leukocytes

(2) Decreased glucose levels

(3) Increased protein levels

2. Viral meningitis is also known as aseptic meningitis. It is characterized clinically by fever, headache, nuchal rigidity, and Kernig's sign.

a. Common causes. Many viruses are associated with viral meningitis, including mumps, echovirus, Coxsackie virus, Epstein-Barr virus, and herpes simplex type 2.

b. CSF findings

(1) Numerous lymphocytes

(2) Normal glucose levels

(3) Moderately increased protein levels

II. VENTRICULAR SYSTEM

A. The **choroid plexus** is a specialized structure that projects into the lateral, third, and fourth ventricles of the brain. It consists of infoldings of blood vessels of the pia mater that are covered by modified ciliated ependymal cells. It secretes the CSF. Tight junctions of the choroid plexus cells form the blood-CSF barrier.

B. Ventricles contain CSF and choroid plexus.

1. The two **lateral ventricles** communicate with the third ventricle through the interventricular **foramina of Monro.**

2. The **third ventricle** is located between the medial walls of the diencephalon. It communicates with the fourth ventricle through the cerebral aqueduct.

3. The **cerebral aqueduct** connects the third and fourth ventricles. It has no choroid plexus. Blockage of the cerebral aqueduct results in hydrocephalus.

4. The **fourth ventricle** communicates with the subarachnoid space through three outlet foramina: lateral foramina of Luschka (2) and medial foramen of Magendie (1).

C. Hydrocephalus is dilation of the cerebral ventricles caused by blockage of the CSF pathways. It is characterized by excessive accumulation of CSF in the cerebral ventricles or subarachnoid space.

1. Noncommunicating hydrocephalus results from obstruction within the ventricles (e.g., congenital aqueductal stenosis).

2. Communicating hydrocephalus results from blockage within the subarachnoid space (e.g., adhesions after meningitis).

3. Normal-pressure hydrocephalus occurs when the CSF is not absorbed by the arachnoid villi. It may occur secondary to posttraumatic meningeal hemorrhage. Clinically, it is characterized by the triad of progressive dementia, ataxic gait, and urinary incontinence. **(Remember: wacky, wobbly, and wet.)**

4. Hydrocephalus ex vacuo results from a loss of cells in the caudate nucleus (e.g., Huntington's disease).

5. Pseudotumor cerebri (benign intracranial hypertension) results from increased resistance to CSF outflow at the arachnoid villi. It occurs in obese young women and is characterized by papilledema without mass, elevated CSF pressure, and deteriorating vision. The ventricles may be slit-like.

III. CEREBROSPINAL FLUID is a colorless acellular fluid. It flows through the ventricles and into the subarachnoid space.

A. Function

1. CSF supports the central nervous system (CNS) and protects it against concussive injury.

2. It **transports hormones** and hormone-releasing factors.

3. It **removes metabolic waste products** through absorption.

B. Formation and absorption. CSF is formed by the choroid plexus. Absorption is primarily through the arachnoid villi into the superior sagittal sinus.

C. The composition of CSF is clinically relevant (Table 2-1).

1. The normal number of **mononuclear cells** is less than $5/\mu l$.

Table 2-1
Cerebrospinal Fluid Profiles in Subarachnoid Hemorrhage, Bacterial Meningitis, and Viral Encephalitis

Cerebrospinal Fluid	Normal	Subarachnoid Hemorrhage	Bacterial Meningitis	Viral Encephalitis
Color	Clear	Bloody	Cloudy	Clear, cloudy
Cell count/mm^3	< 5 lymphocytes	Red blood cells present	> 1000 poly-morphonuclear leukocytes	25–500 lymphocytes
Protein	< 45 mg/dl	Normal to slightly elevated	Elevated >100 mg/dl	Slightly elevated < 100 mg/dl
Glucose ~ 66% of blood (80–120 mg/dl)	> 45 mg/dl	Normal	Reduced	Normal

Cell counts in infants < 10 cells/mm^3; protein in infants = 20–170 mg/dl.

2. **Red blood cells** in the CSF indicate subarachnoid hemorrhage (e.g., caused by trauma or a ruptured berry aneurysm).

3. **CSF glucose** levels are normally 50 to 75 mg/dl (66% of the blood glucose level). Glucose levels are normal in patients with viral meningitis and decreased in patients with bacterial meningitis.

4. **Total protein levels** are normally between 15 and 45 mg/dl in the lumbar cistern. Protein levels are increased in patients with bacterial meningitis and normal or slightly increased in patients with viral meningitis.

5. **Normal CSF pressure** in the lateral recumbent position ranges from 80 to 180 mm H_2O. Brain tumors and meningitis elevate CSF pressure.

IV. HERNIATION (Figures 2-2, 2-3, 2-4, 2-5, 2-6, and 2-7)

A. **Transtentorial (uncal) herniation** is protrusion of the brain through the tentorial incisure.

B. **Transforaminal (tonsillar) herniation** is protrusion of the brain stem and cerebellum through the foramen magnum.

C. **Subfalcial herniation** is herniation below the falx cerebri.

Figure 2-2.   Coronal section of a tumor in the supratentorial compartment. (*1*) Anterior cerebral artery; (*2*) subfalcial herniation; (*3*) shifting of ventricles; (*4*) posterior cerebral artery (compression results in contralateral hemianopia); (*5*) uncal (transtentorial) herniation; (*6*) Kernohan's notch, with damaged corticospinal and corticobulbar fibers; (*7*) tentorium cerebelli; (*8*) pyramidal cells that give rise to the corticospinal tract; (*9*) tonsillar (transforaminal) herniation, which damages vital medullary centers. (Adapted with permission from Leech RW, Shumann RM: *Neuropathology.* New York, Harper & Row, 1982, p. 16.)

Figure 2-3. Axial section through the midbrain and the herniating parahippocampal gyrus. The left oculo-motor nerve is being stretched (dilated pupil). The left posterior cerebral artery is compressed, resulting in a contralateral hemianopia. The right crus cerebri is damaged (Kernohan's notch) by the free edge of the tentorial incisure, resulting in a contralateral hemiparesis. Kernohan's notch results in a false localizing sign. The caudal displacement of the brain stem causes rupture of the paramedian arteries of the basilar artery. Hemorrhage into the midbrain and rostral pontine tegmentum is usually fatal (Duret hemorrhages). The posterior cerebral arteries lie superior to the oculomotor nerves. (1) Parahippocampal gyrus; (2) crus cerebri; (3) posterior cerebral artery; (4) optic nerve; (5) optic chiasma; oculomotor nerve; (7) free edge of tentorium; (8) Kernohan's notch. (Adapted with permission from Leech RW, Shumann RM: *Neuropathology*. New York, Harper & Row, 1982, p. 19.)

Figure 2-4. Magnetic resonance imaging scan showing brain trauma. (A) Internal capsule; (B) subdural hematoma; (C) subdural hematoma; (D) thalamus; (E) epidural hematoma. Epidural hematomas may cross dural attachments. Subdural hematomas do not cross dural attachments. The hyperintense signals are caused by methemoglobin. This is a T1-weighted image.

Figure 2-5. Computed tomography scan axial section showing an intraparenchymal hemorrhage in the left frontal lobe. (A) Intraparenchymal hemorrhage; (B) lateral ventricle; (C) internal capsule; (D) calcified glomus in the trigone region of the lateral ventricle.

Figure 2-6.   Computed tomography axial section showing an epidural hematoma and a skull fracture. (*A*) Epidural hematoma; (*B*) skull fracture; (*C*) calcified pineal gland; (*D*) calcified glomus in the trigone region of the lateral ventricle. The epidural hematoma is a classic biconvex, or lentiform, shape.

Figure 2-7.   Computed tomography, axial section, showing a skull fracture (*A*) on the left side. An epidural hematoma (*B*) underlies the fracture. The CT scan shows a bone window.

3

Blood Supply

I. **THE SPINAL CORD AND LOWER BRAIN STEM** are supplied with blood through the **anterior spinal artery** (Figure 3-1).

   A. The anterior spinal artery supplies the **anterior two-thirds of the spinal cord**.

   B. In the **medulla,** the anterior spinal artery supplies the pyramid, medial lemniscus, and root fibers of cranial nerve (CN) XII.

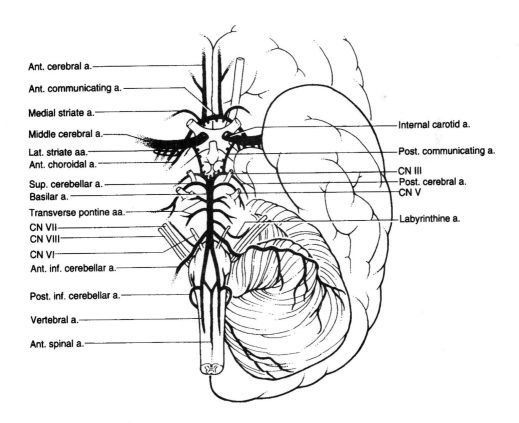

Figure 3-1. Arteries of the base of the brain and brain stem, including the arterial circle of Willis.

II. THE INTERNAL CAROTID SYSTEM (see Figure 3-1) consists of the **internal carotid artery** and its branches.

   A. The **ophthalmic artery** enters the orbit with the optic nerve (CN II). The **central artery of the retina** is a branch of the ophthalmic artery. Occlusion results in blindness.

   B. The **posterior communicating artery** irrigates the hypothalamus and ventral thalamus. An **aneurysm** of this artery is the second most common aneurysm of the circle of Willis. It commonly results in **third-nerve palsy**.

   C. The **anterior choroidal artery** arises from the internal carotid artery. It is not part of the circle of Willis. It perfuses the lateral geniculate body, globus pallidus, and posterior limb of the internal capsule.

   D. The **anterior cerebral artery** (Figure 3-2) supplies the medial surface of the hemisphere from the frontal pole to the parieto-occipital sulcus.

   1. The anterior cerebral artery **irrigates** the **paracentral lobule,** which contains the **leg-foot area of the motor and sensory cortices**.

   2. The **anterior communicating artery** connects the two anterior cerebral arteries. It is the most common site of **aneurysm** of the circle of Willis, which may cause **bitemporal lower quadrantanopia**.

   3. The **medial striate arteries** (see Figure 3-1) are the penetrating arteries of the anterior cerebral artery. They supply the anterior portion of the putamen and caudate nucleus and the anteroinferior part of the internal capsule.

   E. The **middle cerebral artery** (see Figure 3-2)

   1. This artery supplies the lateral convexity of the hemisphere, including:

   a. Broca's and Wernicke's speech areas

   b. The face and arm areas of the motor and sensory cortices

   c. The frontal eye field

A

B

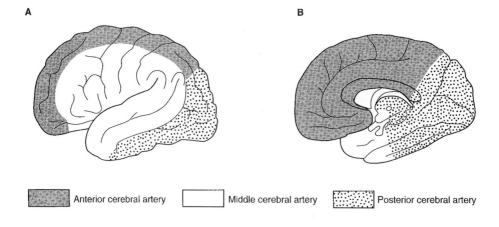

▓▓ Anterior cerebral artery   ☐ Middle cerebral artery   ⁘⁘ Posterior cerebral artery

Figure 3-2.   Cortical territories of the three cerebral arteries. (A) Lateral aspect of the hemisphere. Most of the lateral convexity is supplied by the middle cerebral artery. (B) Medial and inferior aspects of the hemisphere. The anterior cerebral artery supplies the medial surface of the hemisphere from the lamina terminalis to the cuneus. The posterior cerebral artery supplies the visual cortex and the posterior inferior surface of the temporal lobe. (Modified from Töndury, as presented in Sobotta J: *Atlas der Anatomie des Menschen.* Munich, Urban & Schwarzenberg, 1962, pp. 137–138.)

Medial side

Figure 3-3. Coronal section through the cerebral hemisphere at the level of the internal capsule and thalamus showing the major vascular territories.

  2. The **lateral striate arteries** (Figure 3-3) are the penetrating branches of the middle cerebral artery. They are the arteries of **stroke,** and they supply the **internal capsule, caudate nucleus, putamen,** and **globus pallidus.**

III. THE VERTIBROBASILAR SYSTEM (see Figure 3-1)

  A. The **vertebral artery** is a branch of the subclavian artery. It gives rise to the **anterior spinal artery** (see I) and the **posterior inferior cerebellar artery (PICA),** which supplies the dorsolateral quadrant of the medulla. This quadrant includes the nucleus ambiguus (CN IX, X, and XI) and the inferior surface of the cerebellum.

  B. The **basilar artery** is formed by the two vertebral arteries. It gives rise to the following arteries.

   1. The paramedian branches of the **pontine arteries** supply the base of the pons, which includes the corticospinal fibers and the exiting root fibers of the abducent nerve (CN VI).

   2. The **labyrinthine artery** arises from the basilar artery in 15% of people. It arises from the anterior inferior cerebellar artery in 85% of people.

   3. The **anterior inferior cerebellar artery (AICA)** supplies the caudal lateral pontine tegmentum, including CN VII, the spinal trigeminal tract of CN V, and the inferior surface of the cerebellum.

4. The **superior cerebellar artery** supplies the dorsolateral tegmentum of the rostral pons (i.e., rostral to the motor nucleus of CN V), the superior cerebellar peduncle, the superior surface of the cerebellum and cerebellar nuclei, and the cochlear nuclei.

5. The **posterior cerebral artery** (see Figures 3-1, 3-2, and 3-3) is connected to the carotid artery through the posterior communicating artery. It provides the **major blood supply to the midbrain**. It also supplies the thalamus, lateral and medial geniculate bodies, and occipital lobe (which includes the visual cortex and the inferior surface of the temporal lobe, including the hippocampal formation). **Occlusion** of this artery results in a **contralateral hemianopia with macular sparing**.

IV. THE BLOOD SUPPLY OF THE INTERNAL CAPSULE comes primarily from the **lateral striate arteries** of the middle cerebral artery and the **anterior choroidal artery**.

V. VEINS OF THE BRAIN

   A. The **superior cerebral ("bridging") veins** drain into the superior sagittal sinus. Laceration results in a **subdural hematoma**.

   B. The **great cerebral vein of Galen** drains the deep cerebral veins into the **straight sinus**.

VI. VENOUS DURAL SINUSES

   A. The **superior sagittal sinus** receives the bridging veins, and through the arachnoid villi, the cerebrospinal fluid (CSF).

   B. The **cavernous sinus** contains CN III, IV, V-1 and V-2, VI, and the postganglionic sympathetic fibers. It also contains the siphon of the internal carotid artery (Figure 3-4).

Figure 3-4. Magnetic resonance angiogram, lateral projection, showing the major venous sinuses and arteries. Note the bridging veins entering the superior sagittal sinus. *ICA* = internal carotid artery; *MCA* = middle cerebral artery; *PCA* = posterior cerebral artery.

List of structures:

1. Anterior cerebral artery
2. Anterior choroidal artery
3. Anterior inferior cerebellar artery
4. Basilar artery
5. Calcarine artery (of posterior cerebral artery)
6. Callosomarginal artery (of anterior cerebral artery)
7. Callosomarginal and pericallosal arteries
   (of anterior cerebral artery)
8. Internal carotid artery
9. Lateral striate arteries (of middle cerebral artery)

10. Middle cerebral artery
11. Ophthalmic artery
12. Pericallosal artery (of anterior cerebral artery)
13. Posterior cerebral artery
14. Posterior choroidal arteries
    (of posteior cerebral artery)
15. Posterior communicating artery
16. Posterior inferior cerebellar artery
17. Superior cerebellar artery
18. Vertebral artery

Figure 3-5.   (A) Carotid angiogram, lateral projection. (B) Carotid angiogram, anteroposterior projection. (C) Vertebral angiogram, lateral projection. (D) Vertebral angiogram, anteroposterior projection.

VII. ANGIOGRAPHY

A. Carotid angiography. Figures 3-5A and B show the internal carotid artery, anterior cerebral artery, and middle cerebral artery.

B. Vertebral angiography. Figures 3-5C and D show the vertebral artery, PICA and AICA, basilar artery, superior cerebellar artery, and posterior cerebral artery (Figures 3-6 and 3-7).

Figure 3-6.   Arterial anatomy of an MR section; axial (A), sagittal (B, C), coronal (C). Abbreviations: ACAcm = anterior anterior cerebral artery, callosal marginal branch; A2 and A1 are branches of the anterior cerebral artery: ACApc = pericallosal branch of the anterior cerebral artery; ACoA = anterior communicating artery; M1 and M2 are segments of the middle cerebral artery (MCA); MCAb = bifurcation; ICAs = internal carotid artery siphon; PAC = posterior cerebral arterior, PCoA = posterior communicating artery; BA = basilar artery; SCA = superior cerebellar artery. (Reprinted with permission from Grossman CB: *Magenetic Resonance Imaging and Computed Tomography of the Head and Spine,* 2nd ed. Philadelphia, Williams & Wilkins, 1996, p. 124.)

Figure 3-7.   Venous anatomy of an MR section; midsagittal (A), lateral (B), submental-vertex (C). Abbreviations: IhV = interhemispheric veins; SSS = superior sagittal sinus; ISS = inferior sagittal sinus; TsV = thalmostriate veins; StS = straight sinus; PcCbV = precentral cerebellar vein; To = torcula; VG = vein of anterior pontomesencephalic veins. (Reprinted with permission from Grossman CB: *Magenetic Resonance Imaging and Computed Tomography of the Head and Spine*, 2nd ed. Philadelphia, Williams & Wilkins, 1996, p. 125.)

    C. Veins and dural sinuses. Figure 3-8 shows the internal cerebral vein, superior cerebral veins, great cerebral vein, superior ophthalmic vein, and major dural sinuses.

    D. Digital subtraction angiography. See Figures 3-9, 3-10, 3-11, and 3-12.

VIII. THE MIDDLE MENINGEAL ARTERY, a branch of the **maxillary artery,** enters the cranium through the **foramen spinosum**. It supplies most of the dura, including its calvarial portion. Laceration results in **epidural hemorrhage** (hematoma) [Figures 3-13 and 3-14].

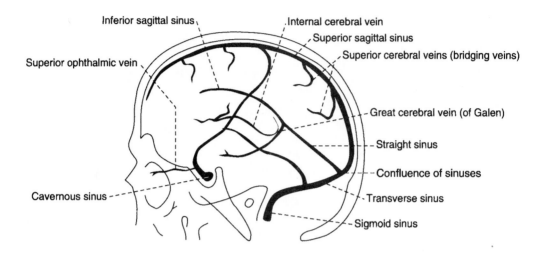

Figure 3-8. Carotid angiogram, venous phase, showing the cerebral veins and venous sinuses.

Figure 3-9. Carotid angiogram, lateral projection. Identify the cortical branches of the anterior cerebral artery (ACA) and middle cerebral artery (MCA). Follow the course of the internal carotid artery (ICA). Remember that aneurysms of the posterior communicating artery may result in third-nerve palsy. The paracentral lobule is irrigated by the callosomarginal artery. Cortical branches of the MCA are designated with dots. PCoM = posterior communicating artery.

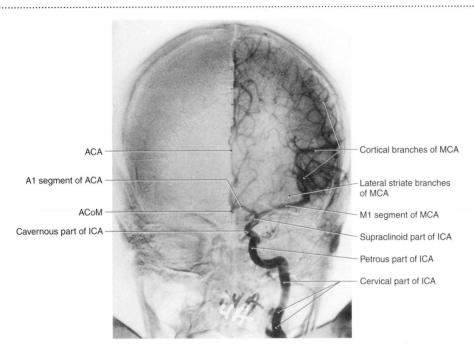

ACA

A1 segment of ACA

ACoM

Cavernous part of ICA

Cortical branches of MCA

Lateral striate branches
of MCA

M1 segment of MCA

Supraclinoid part of ICA

Petrous part of ICA

Cervical part of ICA

Figure 3-10. Carotid angiogram, anteroposterior projection. Identify the anterior cerebral artery (ACA), middle cerebral artery (MCA), and internal carotid artery (ICA). The horizontal branches of the MCA perfuse the basal ganglia and internal capsule. ACoM = anterior communicating artery.

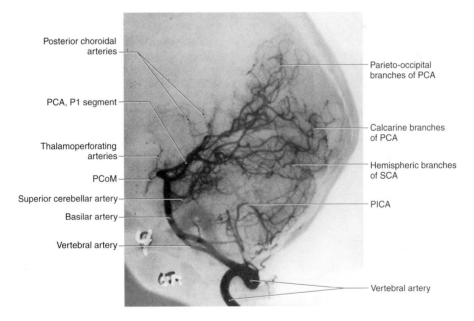

Posterior choroidal
arteries

PCA, P1 segment

Thalamoperforating
arteries

PCoM

Superior cerebellar artery

Basilar artery

Vertebral artery

Parieto-occipital
branches of PCA

Calcarine branches
of PCA

Hemispheric branches
of SCA

PICA

Vertebral artery

Figure 3-11. Vertebral angiogram, lateral projection. Two structures are found between the posterior cerebral artery (PCA) and the superior cerebellar artery: the tentorium and the third cranial nerve. PCoM = posterior communicating artery; PICA = posterior inferior cerebellar artery; SCA = superior cerebellar artery.

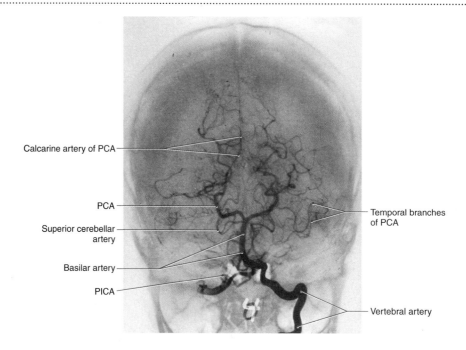

Figure 3-12.   Vertebral angiogram, anteroposterior projection. Which artery supplies the visual cortex? The calcarine artery, a branch of the posterior cerebral artery (*PCA*). Occlusion of the PCA (calcarine artery) results in a contralateral homonymous hemianopia, with macular sparing. *PICA* = posterior inferior cerebellar artery.

Figure 3-13.   An epidural hematoma results from laceration of the middle meningeal artery. Arterial bleeding into the epidural space forms a biconvex clot. The classic "lucid interval" is seen in 50% of cases. Skull fractures are usually found. Epidural hematomas rarely cross sutural lines. (Reprinted with permission from Osburn AG, Tong KA: *Handbook of Neuroradiology: Brain and Skull.* St. Louis, Mosby, 1996, p. 191.)

Figure 3-14.   A subdural hematoma (SDH) results from lacerated bridging veins. SDHs are frequently accompanied by traumatic subarachnoid hemorrhages and cortical contusions. Sudden deceleration of the head causes tearing of the superior cerebral veins. The SDH extends over the crest of the convexity into the interhemispheric fissure, but does not cross the dural attachment of the falx cerebri. The clot can be crescent-shaped, biconvex, or multiloculated. SDHs are more common than epidural hematomas. SDHs always cause brain damage. (Reprinted with permission from Osburn AG, Tong KA: *Handbook of Neuroradiology: Brain and Skull.* St. Louis, Mosby, 1996, p. 192.)

4
Development of the Nervous System

I. THE NEURAL TUBE (Figure 4-1) gives rise to the **central nervous system (CNS)** [i.e., brain and spinal cord.]

   A. The **brain stem** and spinal cord have:

      1. An **alar plate** that gives rise to the **sensory neurons**

      2. A **basal plate** that gives rise to the **motor neurons** (Figure 4-2)

   B. The neural tube gives rise to **three primary vesicles,** which develop into **five secondary vesicles** (Figure 4-3).

   C. Alpha-fetoprotein (AFP) is found in the amniotic fluid and maternal serum. It is an indicator of neural tube defects (e.g., spina bifida, anencephaly). AFP levels are reduced in mothers of fetuses with Down syndrome.

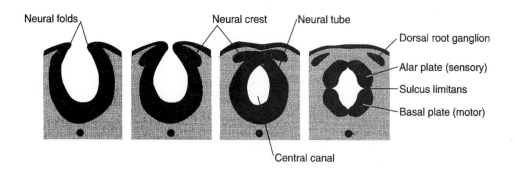

Figure 4-1. Development of the neural tube and crest. The alar plate gives rise to sensory neurons. The basal plate gives rise to motor neurons. The neural crest gives rise to the peripheral nervous system.

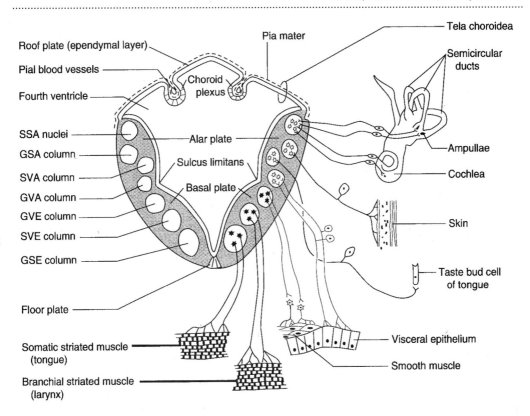

Figure 4-2.   The brain stem showing the cell columns derived from the alar and basal plates. The seven cranial nerve modalities are shown. GSA = general somatic afferent; GSE = general somatic efferent; GVA = general visceral afferent; GVE = general visceral efferent; SSA = special somatic afferent; SVA = special visceral afferent; SVE = special visceral efferent. (Adapted with permission from Patten BM: *Human Embryology*, 3rd ed. New York, McGraw-Hill, 1969, p. 298.)

II. THE NEURAL CREST (see Figure 4-1) gives rise to:

   A. The **peripheral nervous system (PNS)** [i.e., peripheral nerves and sensory and autonomic ganglia]

   B. The following cells:

   1. Pseudounipolar ganglion cells of the spinal and cranial nerve ganglia

   2. Schwann cells (which elaborate the myelin sheath)

   3. Multipolar ganglion cells of autonomic ganglia

   4. Leptomeninges (the pia-arachnoid) envelop the brain and spinal cord

   5. Chromaffin cells of the suprarenal medulla (which elaborate epinephrine)

   6. Pigment cells (melanocytes)

   7. Odontoblasts (which elaborate predentin)

   8. Aorticopulmonary septum of the **heart**

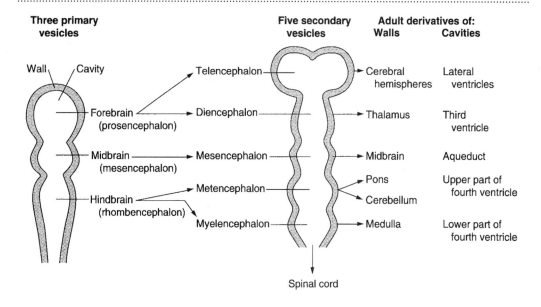

Figure 4-3. The brain vesicles indicating the adult derivatives of their walls and cavities. (Reprinted with permission from Moore KL: *The Developing Human: Clinically Orienting Embryology*, 4th ed. Philadelphia, WB Saunders, 1988, p. 380.)

   9. Parafollicular cells (calcitonin-producing C-cells)

   10. Skeletal and **connective tissue components** of the **pharyngeal arches**

III. THE ANTERIOR NEUROPORE. The closure of the anterior neuropore gives rise to the lamina terminalis. **Failure to close results in anencephaly** (i.e., failure of the brain to develop).

IV. THE POSTERIOR NEUROPORE. Failure to close results in spina bifida (Figure 4-4).

V. MICROGLIA arise from the monocytes.

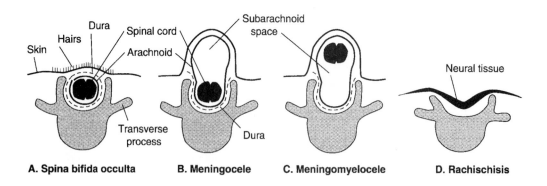

A. Spina bifida occulta   **B. Meningocele**   **C. Meningomyelocele**   **D. Rachischisis**

Figure 4-4. The various types of spina bifida. (Reprinted with permission from Sadler TW: *Langman's Medical Embryology*, 6th ed. Baltimore, Williams & Wilkins, 1990, p. 363.)

VI. MYELINATION begins in the fourth month of gestation. Myelination of the corticospinal tracts is not completed until the end of the second postnatal year, when the tracts become functional. Myelination in the cerebral association cortex continues into the third decade.

  A. **Myelination of the CNS** is accomplished by oligodendrocytes, which are not found in the retina.

  B. **Myelination of the PNS** is accomplished by Schwann cells (Figures 4-5A, B).

VII. POSITIONAL CHANGES OF THE SPINAL CORD

  A. In the **newborn,** the conus medullaris ends at the third lumbar vertebra (L-3).

  B. In the **adult,** the conus medullaris ends at L-1.

VIII. THE OPTIC NERVE AND CHIASMA are derived from the diencephalon. The optic nerve fibers occupy the **choroid fissure**. Failure of this fissure to close results in **coloboma iridis**.

IX. THE HYPOPHYSIS (pituitary gland) is derived from two embryologic substrata (Figures 4-6 and 4-7).

  A. **Adenohypophysis** is derived from an ectodermal diverticulum of the primitive mouth cavity (stomodeum), which is also called **Rathke's pouch**. Remnants of Rathke's pouch may give rise to a congenital cystic tumor, a **craniopharyngioma**.

  B. **Neurohypophysis** develops from a ventral evagination of the hypothalamus (neuroectoderm of the neural tube).

X. CONGENITAL MALFORMATIONS OF THE CNS

  A. **Anencephaly (meroanencephaly)** results from failure of the anterior neuropore to close. As a result, the brain does not develop. The frequency of this condition is 1:1000.

  B. **Spina bifida** results from failure of the posterior neuropore to form. The defect usually occurs in the sacrolumbar region. The frequency of spina bifida occulta is 10%.

  C. **Cranium bifidum** results from a defect in the occipital bone through which meninges, cerebellar tissure, and the fourth ventricle may herniate.

  D. **Arnold-Chiari** malformation (type 2) has a frequency of 1:1000 (Figure 4-8).

  E. **Dandy-Walker** malformation has a frequency of 1:25000. It may result from riboflavin inhibitors, posterior fossa trauma, or viral infection (Figure 4-9).

  F. **Hydrocephalus** is most commonly caused by stenosis of the cerebral aqueduct during development. Excessive cerebrospinal fluid accumulates in the ventricles and subarachnoid space. This condition may result from maternal infection (cytomegalovirus and toxoplasmosis). The frequency is 1:1000.

  G. **Fetal alcohol syndrome** is the most common cause of mental retardation. It includes microcephaly and congenital heart disease; holoprosencephaly is the most severe manifestation.

  H. **Holoprosencephaly** results from failure of midline cleavage of the embyonic forebrain. The telenceplalon contains a singular ventricular cavity; is seen in trisomy 13 (Patau syndrome); the corpus callosum may be absent; holoprosencephaly is the most severe manifestation of the fetal alcohol syndrome.

  I. **Hydranencephaly** results from bilateral hemispheric infarction secondary to occlusion of the carotid arteries. The hemispheres are replaced by hugely dilated ventricles.

Figure 4-5.   Myelination in the pyramids and in the middle cerebellar peduncles. (A) 9 months old; myelination incomplete. (B) 50-year-old adult; myelination is complete in all systems. (Reprinted with permission from Haymaker W, Adams RD: *Histology and Histopathology of the Nervous System*. Springfield, Charles C Thomas, 1982, p. 169.)

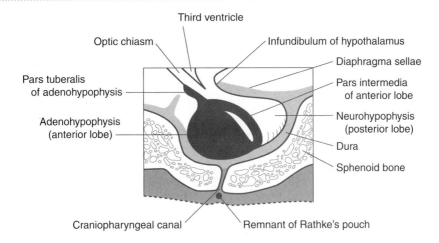

Figure 4-6. Midsagittal section through the hypophysis and sella turcica. The adenohypophysis, including the pars tuberalis and pars intermedia, is derived from Rathke's pouch (oroectoderm). The neurohypophysis arises from the infundibulum of the hypothalamus (neuroectoderm).

Figure 4-7. Midsagittal section through the brain stem and diencephalon. A craniopharyngioma (*arrows*) lies suprasellar in the midline. It compresses the optic chiasm and hypothalamus. This tumor is the most common supratentorial tumor that occurs in childhood and the most common cause of hypopituitarism in children. This is a T1-weighted magnetic resonance imaging scan.

A — Foramen magnum

B

Figure 4-8. Arnold-Chiari malformation. Midsagittal section. (A) Normal cerebellum, fourth ventricle, and brain stem. (B) Abnormal cerebellum, fourth ventricle, and brain stem showing the common congenital anomalies: (*1*) beaking of the tectal plate, (*2*) aqueductal stenosis, (*3*) kinking and transforaminal herniation of the medulla into the vertebral canal, and (*4*) herniation and unrolling of the cerebellar vermis into the vertebral canal. An accompanying meningomyelocele is common. (Reprinted with permission from Fix JD: *BRS Neuroanatomy*. Baltimore, Williams & Wilkins, 1996, p. 72.)

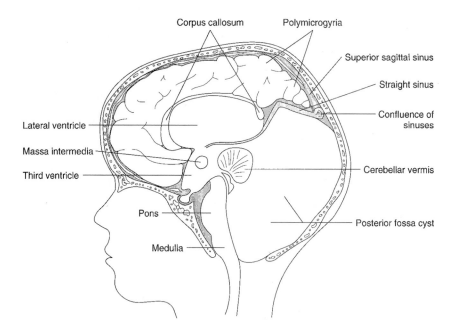

Figure 4-9. Dandy-Walker malformation. Midsagittal section. An enormous dilation of the fourth ventricle results from failure of the foramina of Luschka and Magendie to open. This condition is associated with occipital meningocele, elevation of the confluence of the sinuses (torcular Herophili), agenesis of the cerebellar vermis, and splenium of the corpus callosum. (Reprinted with permission from Dudek RW, Fix JD: *BRS Embryology*. Baltimore, Williams & Wilkins, 1997, p. 97.)

5

Neurohistology

I. NEURONS are classified by the number of processes (Figure 5-1).

   A. Pseudounipolar neurons are located in the spinal dorsal root ganglia and sensory ganglia of cranial nerves (CN) V, VII, IX, and X.

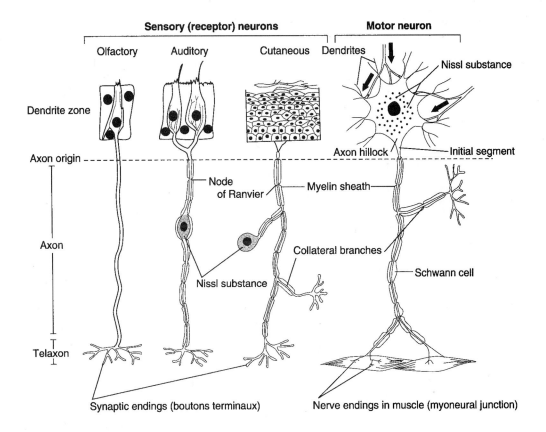

Figure 5-1. Types of nerve cells. Olfactory neurons are bipolar and unmyelinated. Auditory neurons are bipolar and myelinated. Dorsal root ganglion cells (cutaneous) are pseudounipolar and myelinated. Motor neurons are multipolar and myelinated. *Arrows* indicate input through the axons of other neurons. Nerve cells are characterized by the presence of Nissl substance and rough endoplasmic reticulum. (Modified with permission from Carpenter MB, Sutin J: *Human Neuroanatomy.* Baltimore, Williams & Wilkins, 1983, p. 92.)

B. Bipolar neurons are found in the cochlear and vestibular ganglia of CN VIII, in the olfactory nerve (CN I), and in the retina.

C. Multipolar neurons are the largest population of nerve cells in the nervous system. This group includes motor neurons, neurons of the autonomic nervous system, interneurons, pyramidal cells of the cerebral cortex, and Purkinje's cells of the cerebellar cortex.

D. There are approximately 10^{11} neurons in the brain and approximately 10^{10} neurons in the neocortex.

II. NISSL SUBSTANCE is characteristic of neurons. It consists of rosettes of polysomes and rough endoplasmic reticulum; therefore, it has a role in protein synthesis. Nissl substance is found in the **nerve cell body (perikaryon)** and **dendrites,** not in the axon hillock or axon.

III. AXONAL TRANSPORT mediates the intracellular distribution of secretory proteins, organelles, and cytoskeletal elements. It is inhibited by colchicine, which depolymerizes microtubules.

A. Fast anterograde axonal transport is responsible for transporting all newly synthesized membranous organelles (vesicles) and precursors of neurotransmitters. This process occurs at the rate of 200 to 400 mm/day. It is mediated by neurotubules and **kinesin.** (Fast transport is neurotubule-dependent.)

B. Slow anterograde transport is responsible for transporting fibrillar cytoskeletal and protoplasmic elements. This process occurs at the rate of 1 to 5 mm/day.

C. Fast retrograde transport returns used materials from the axon terminal to the cell body for degradation and recycling at a rate of 100 to 200 mm/day. It transports **nerve growth factor, neurotropic viruses,** and toxins, such as **herpes simplex, rabies, poliovirus,** and **tetanus toxin**. It is mediated by neurotubules and **dynein.**

IV. WALLERIAN DEGENERATION is anterograde degeneration characterized by the disappearance of axons and myelin sheaths and the secondary proliferation of Schwann cells. It occurs in the central nervous system (CNS) and the peripheral nervous system (PNS).

V. CHROMATOLYSIS is the result of retrograde degeneration in the neurons of the CNS and PNS. There is a loss of Nissl substance after axotomy.

VI. REGENERATION OF NERVE CELLS

A. CNS. Effective regeneration does not occur in the CNS. For example, there is no regeneration of the optic nerve, which is a tract of the diencephalon. There are no basement membranes or endoneural investments surrounding the axons of the CNS.

B. PNS. Regeneration does occur in the PNS. The proximal tip of a severed axon grows into the endoneural tube, which consists of Schwann cell basement membrane and endoneurium. The axon sprout grows at the rate of 3 mm/day (Figure 5-2).

VII. GLIAL CELLS are the nonneural cells of the nervous system.

A. Macroglia consist of **astrocytes and oligodendrocytes.**

1. Astrocytes perform the following functions:

a. They project foot processes that envelop the basement membrane of capillaries, neurons, and synapses.

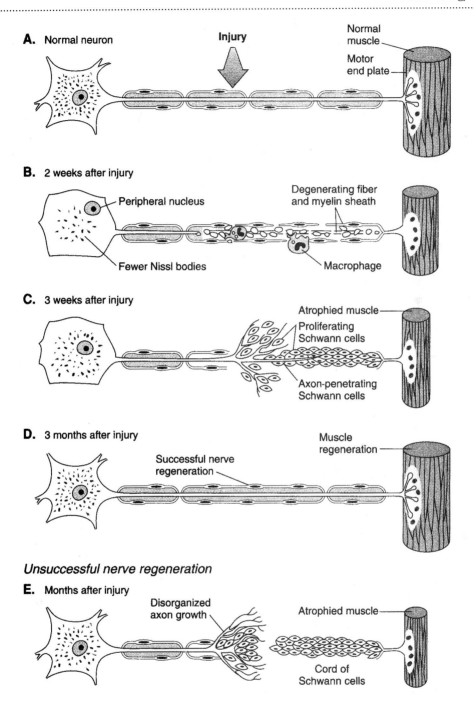

A. Normal neuron

Injury

Normal muscle

Motor end plate

B. 2 weeks after injury

Peripheral nucleus

Degenerating fiber and myelin sheath

Fewer Nissl bodies

Macrophage

C. 3 weeks after injury

Atrophied muscle

Proliferating Schwann cells

Axon-penetrating Schwann cells

D. 3 months after injury

Successful nerve regeneration

Muscle regeneration

Unsuccessful nerve regeneration

E. Months after injury

Disorganized axon growth

Atrophied muscle

Cord of Schwann cells

Figure 5-2.   Schematic diagram of peripheral nerve regeneration.

    b. They form the external and internal glial-limiting membranes of the CNS.

    c. They play a role in the metabolism of certain neurotransmitters [e.g., γ-amino-butyric acid (GABA), serotonin, glutamate].

    d. They buffer the potassium concentration of the extracellular space.

    e. They form glial scars in damaged areas of the brain (i.e., astrogliosis).

    f. They contain glial fibrillary acidic protein (GFAP), which is a marker for astrocytes.

    g. They contain glutamine synthetase, another biochemical marker for astrocytes.

    h. May be identified with monoclonal antibodies (e.g., A_2B_5).

  2. **Oligodendrocytes** are the myelin-forming cells of the CNS. One oligodendrocyte can myelinate as many as 30 axons.

B. **Microglia** arise from monocytes and function as the scavenger cells (phagocytes) of the CNS.

C. **Ependymal cells** are ciliated cells that line the central canal and ventricles of the brain. They also line the luminal surface of the choroid plexus. These cells **produce cerebrospinal fluid (CSF).**

D. **Tanycytes** are modified ependymal cells that contact capillaries and neurons. They mediate cellular transport between the ventricles and the neuropil. They project to hypothalamic nuclei that regulate the release of gonadotropic hormone from the adenohypophysis.

E. **Schwann cells** are derived from the neural crest. They are the myelin-forming cells of the PNS. One Schwann cell can myelinate only one internode. Schwann cells invest all myelinated and unmyelinated axons of the PNS and are separated from each other by the **nodes of Ranvier.**

VIII. **THE BLOOD–BRAIN BARRIER** consists of the tight junctions of nonfenestrated endothelial cells; some authorities include the astrocytic foot processes. **Infarction of brain tissue** destroys the tight junctions of endothelial cells and results in **vasogenic edema,** which is an infiltrate of plasma into the extracellular space.

IX. **THE BLOOD–CSF BARRIER** consists of the tight junctions between the cuboidal epithelial cells of the choroid plexus. The barrier is permeable to some circulating peptides (e.g., insulin) and plasma proteins (e.g., prealbumin).

X. **PIGMENTS AND INCLUSIONS**

A. **Lipofuscin granules** are pigmented cytoplasmic inclusions that commonly accumulate with aging. They are considered residual bodies that are derived from lysosomes.

B. **Melanin (neuromelanin)** is blackish intracytoplasmic pigment found in the substantia nigra and locus coeruleus. It disappears from nigral neurons in patients who have Parkinson's disease.

C. **Lewy bodies** are neuronal inclusions that are characteristic of Parkinson's disease.

D. **Negri bodies** are intracytoplasmic inclusions that are pathognomonic of rabies. They are found in the pyramidal cells of the hippocampus and the Purkinje cells of the cerebellum.

E. **Hirano bodies** are intraneuronal, eosinophilic, rodlike inclusions that are found in the hippocampus of patients with Alzheimer's disease.

Table 5-1
Classification of Nerve Fibers

Fiber	Diameter (μm)*	Conduction Velocity (m/sec)	Function
Sensory axons			
Ia (A-α)	12–20	70–120	Proprioception, muscle spindles
Ib (A-α)	12–20	70–120	Proprioception, Golgi tendon organs
II (A-β)	5–12	30–70	Touch, pressure, and vibration
III (A-δ)	2–5	12–30	Touch, pressure, fast pain, and temperature
IV (C)	0.5–1	0.5–2	Slow pain and temperature, unmyelinated fibers
Motor axons			
Alpha (A-α)	12–20	15–120	Alpha motor neurons of ventral horn (innervate extrafusal muscle fibers)
Gamma (A-γ)	2–10	10–45	Gamma motor neurons of ventral horn (innervate intrafusal muscle fibers)
Preganglionic autonomic fibers (B)	< 3	3–15	Myelinated preganglionic autonomic fibers
Postganglionic autonomic fibers (C)	1	2	Unmyelinated postganglionic autonomic fibers

*Myelin sheath included if present.

F. Neurofibrillary tangles consist of intracytoplasmic degenerated neurofilaments. They are seen in patients with Alzheimer's disease.

G. Cowdry type A inclusion bodies are intranuclear inclusions that are found in neurons and glia in herpes simplex encephalitis.

XI. THE CLASSIFICATION OF NERVE FIBERS is shown in Table 5-1.

XII. TUMORS OF THE CNS AND PNS are shown in Figure 5-3.

A. One-third of brain tumors are metastatic, and two-thirds are primary. In metastatic tumors, the primary site of malignancy is the lung in 35% of cases, the breast in 17%, in the gastrointestinal tract in 6%, melanoma in 6%, and the kidney in 5%.

B. Brain tumors are classified as glial (50%) or nonglial (50%).

C. According to national board questions, the five most common brain tumors are:

   1. Glioblastoma multiforme, the most common and most fatal type

   2. Meningioma, a benign noninvasive tumor of the falx and the convexity of the hemisphere

   3. Schwannoma, a benign peripheral tumor derived from Schwann cells

   4. Ependymoma, which is found in the ventricles and accounts for 60% of spinal cord gliomas

   5. Medulloblastoma, which is the second most common posterior fossa tumor seen in children and may metastasize through the CSF tracts

D. Neuromagnetic images (NMI) of the brain and brain stems.

A

Germinomas
- germ cell tumors that are commonly seen in the pineal region (>50%)
- overlie the tectum of the midbrain
- cause obstructive hydrocephalus due to aqueductal stenosis
- the common cause of Parinaud's syndrome

Brain abscesses
- may result from sinusitis, mastoiditis, hematogenous spread
- location: frontal and temporal lobes, cerebellum
- organisms: streptococci, staphlococci, and pneumococci
- result in cerebral edema and herniation

Colloid cysts of third ventricle
- comprise 2% of intracranial gliomas
- are of ependymal origin
- found at the interventricular foraminia
- ventricular obstruction results in increased intracranial pressure, and may cause positional headaches, "drop attacks," or sudden death

Meningiomas
- derived from arachnoid cap cells and represent the second most common primary intracranial brain tumor after astrocytomas (15%)
- are not invasive; they indent the brain; may produce hyperostosis
- pathology: concentric whorls and calcified psammoma bodies
- location: parasagittal and convexity
- gender: females > men
- associated with neurofibromatosis-2 (NF-2)

Astrocytomas
- represent 20% of the gliomas
- historically benign
- diffusely infiltrate the hemispheric white matter
- most common glioma found in the posterior fossa of children

Glioblastoma multiforme
- represents 55% of gliomas
- malignant; rapidly fatal astrocytic tumor
- commonly found in the frontal and temporal lobes and basal ganglia
- frequently crosses the midline via the corpus callosum (butterfly glioma)
- most common primary brain tumor
- histology: pseudopalisades, perivascular pseudorosettes

Ependymomas

Oligodendrogliomas
- represent 5% of all the gliomas
- grow slowly and are relatively benign
- most common in the frontal lobe
- calcification in 50% of cases
- cells look like "fried eggs" (perinuclear halos)

B

Choroid plexus papillomas
- historically benign
- represent 2% of the gliomas
- one of the most common brain tumors in patients < 2 years of age
- occur in decreasing frequency: fourth, lateral, and third ventricle
- CSF overproduction may cause hydrocephalus

Cerebellar astrocytomas
- benign tumors of childhood with good prognosis
- most common pediatric intracranial tumor
- contain pilocytic astrocytes and Rosenthal fibers

Medulloblastomas
- represent 7% of primary brain tumors
- represent a primitive neuroectodermal tumor (PNET)
- second most common posterior fossa tumor in children
- responsible for the posterior vermis syndrome
- can metastasize via the CSF tracts
- highly radiosensitive

Hemangioblastomas
- characterized by abundant capillary blood vessels and foamy cells; most often found in the cerebellum
- when found in the cerebellum and retina, may represent a part of the von Hippel-Lindau syndrome
- 2% of primary intracranial tumors; 10% of posterior fossa tumors

Craniopharyngiomas
- represent 3% of primary brain tumors
- derived from epithelial remnants of Rathke's pouch
- location: suprasellar and inferior to the optic chiasma
- cause bitemporal hemianopia and hypopituitarism
- calcification is common

Pituitary adenomas (PA)
- most common tumors of the pituitary gland
- prolactinoma is the most common (PA)
- derived from the stomodeum (Rathke's pouch)
- represent 8% of primary brain tumors
- may cause hypopituitarism, visual field defects (bitemporal hemianopia and cranial nerve palsies CNN III, IV, VI, V-1 and V-2, and postganglionic sympathetic fibers to the dilator muscle of the iris)

Schwannomas (acoustic neuromas)
- consist of Schwann cells and arise from the vestibular division of CN VIII
- compromise approx. 8% of intracranial neoplasms
- pathology: Antoni A and B tissue and Verocay bodies
- bilateral acoustic neuromas are diagnostic of NF-2

Brain stem glioma
- usually a benign pilocytic astrocytoma
- usually causes cranial nerve palsies
- may cause the "locked-in" syndrome

Intraspinal tumors
- Schwannomas 30%
- Meningiomas 25%
- Gliomas 20%
- Sarcomas 12%
- Ependymomas represent 60% of intramedullary gliomas

Ependymomas
- represent 5% of the gliomas
- histology: benign, ependymal tubules, perivascular pseudorosettes
- 40% are supratentorial; 60% are infratentorial (posterior fossa)
- most common spinal cord glioma (60%)
- third most common posterior fossa tumor in children and adolescents

Figure 5-3.   Tumors of the central and peripheral nervous systems. (*A*) Supratentorial tumors. (*B*) Infratentorial (posterior fossa) and intraspinal tumors. In children, 70% of tumors are infratentorial. In adults, 70% of tumors are supratentorial. *CN* = cranial nerve; *CSF* = cerebrospinal fluid.

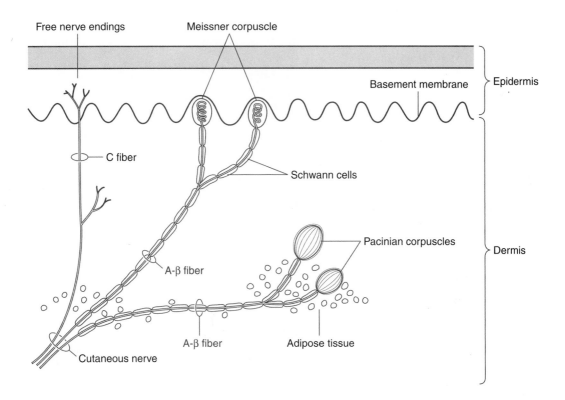

Figure 5-4.   Three important cutaneous receptors. Free nerve endings mediate pain and temperature sensation. Meissner corpuscles of the dermal papillae mediate tactile two-point discrimination. Pacinian corpuscles of the dermis mediate touch, pressure, and vibration sensation. Merkel disks mediate light touch.

XIII. CUTANEOUS RECEPTORS (Figure 5-4) are divided into two large groups: free nerve endings and encapsulated endings.

    A. Free nerve endings are nociceptors (pain) and thermoreceptors (cold and heat).

    B. Encapsulated endings are touch receptors (Meissner's corpuscles) and pressure and vibration receptors (Pacinian corpuscles).

    C. Merkel disks are unencapsulated light touch receptors.

XIV. CASE STUDIES OF BRAIN TUMORS

Case 1.

Astrocytoma (grade II), coronal, TI image, Five-year-old boy presenting with seizures. Temporal lobe epilepsy. A slow growing benign glioma. Arrows point to amorphous thickening of cortical gray.

(Reprinted with permission from Yock DH Jr.: *Magnetic Resonance Imaging of CNS Disease: A Teaching File*, 2nd ed. St. Louis, Mosby, 2002, Case 72.)

Case 2.

Cystic cerebellar astrocytoma, sagittal, T1, 4-year old-girl presenting with clumsiness and headaches. Gliomas of the cerebellum are among the most frequent posterior fossa tumors. These tumors are benign. Arrow points to tumor nodule at margin of cyst.

(Reprinted with permission from Yock DH Jr.: *Magnetic Resonance Imaging of CNS Disease: A Teaching File*, 2nd ed. St. Louis, Mosby, 2002, Case 142.)

Case 3.

Glioblastoma multiforme, axial, T2; 62-year-old female presents with headaches and a left hemiparesis; the most comon glial tumor. Papilldema and herniation are seen. Tumor cells cross the corpus callosum resulting in a "butterfly" glioma; seen in axial and coronal slices.

(Reprinted with permission from Yock DH Jr.: *Magnetic Resonance Imaging of CNS Disease: A Teaching File,* 2nd ed. St. Louis, Mosby, 2002, Case 104.)

Case 4.

Oligodendroglioma, axial, T2, 53-year-old man presenting with severe headache. Oligodendrocytomas show calcification and hemorrhage, more so than astrocytomas. An oligodendrocytoma may become a malignant glioblastoma. They are found most frequently in the temporal lobe (temporal lobe epilepsy). The arrow points to erosion of the inner table.

(Reprinted with permission from Yock DH Jr.: *Magnetic Resonance Imaging of CNS Disease: A Teaching File,* 2nd ed. St. Louis, Mosby, 2002, Case 116.)

Case 5.

Malignant ependymoma, axial, T2, 2-year-old female presenting with nausea and vomiting; large "flow voids" shows a highly vascular lesion (arrows). Periventricular edema is seen along the border of the hydrocephalic right lateral ventricle. Is found in the fourth ventricle more frequently than in the lateral ventricles.

(Reprinted with permission from Yock DH Jr.: *Magnetic Resonance Imaging of CNS Disease: A Teaching File*, 2nd ed. St. Louis, Mosby, 2002, Case 124.)

Case 6.

Meningioma (convexity), parasagittal, T1, 44-year-old woman, presenting with signs of intracranial pressure (e.g., headaches). "Dural tails" are marked with white arrows; tumor shows slow growth and is not invasive.

(Reprinted with permission from Yock DH Jr.: *Magnetic Resonance Imaging of CNS Disease: A Teaching File*, 2nd ed. St. Louis, Mosby, 2002, Case 50.)

Case 7.

Acoustic Schwannoma, axial, T1, 38-year-old woman with ipsilateral hearing loss, tinnitus, and cerebellar ataxia; white arrows show expanded internal auditory meatus; black arrows show cisternal widening. Cranial nerves involved: CNN VII, VIII, and lateral pons (trigeminal spinal tract).

(Reprinted with permission from Yock DH Jr.: *Magnetic Resonance Imaging of CNS Disease: A Teaching File*, 2nd ed. St. Louis, Mosby, 2002, Case 195.)

Case 8.

Meningioma coronal, T1, mass in cerebellopontine angle; 38-year-old woman presents with left facial pain. Tumor may involve cranial nerves: CN V, VII, and VIII (arrow points to normal CN V.)

(Reprinted with permission from Yock DH Jr.: *Magnetic Resonance Imaging of CNS Disease: A Teaching File*, 2nd ed. St. Louis, Mosby, 2002, Case 197.)

Case 9.

Medulloblastoma, coronal, T1, 9-year-old girl presents with ataxia, diplopia and headaches; differential diagnosis includes: astrocytoma, ependymoma, hemangioblastoma, and choroid plexus papilloma. Arise only in the cerebellum.

(Reprinted with permission from Yock DH Jr.: *Magnetic Resonance Imaging of CNS Disease: A Teaching File*, 2nd ed. St. Louis, Mosby, 2002, Case 150.)

Case 10.

Pituitary adenoma, parasagittal, T1, 38-year-old man with blurred vision; white arrowhead shows expanded sella turcica.

(Reprinted with permission from Yock DH Jr.: *Magnetic Resonance Imaging of CNS Disease: A Teaching File*, 2nd ed. St. Louis, Mosby, 2002, Case 225.)

Case 11.

Craniopharyngioma, sagittal, T1, 8-year-old girl presents with headache and weight gain; anosmia with bitemporal hemianopia; they compress chiasm, pituitary gland, and third ventricle; most common of the supratentorial tumors occuring in children; thought to be derived from Rathke's pouch (stomodeum). Arrow points to chiasm.

(Reprinted with permission from Yock DH Jr.: *Magnetic Resonance Imaging of CNS Disease: A Teaching File*, 2nd ed. St. Louis, Mosby, 2002, Case 250.)

Case 12.

Spinal cord ependymoma, sagittal T2, 47-year-old woman presenting with neck and back pain. Ependymomas are the most common intramedullary tumors of the spinal cord.

(Reprinted with permission from Yock DH Jr.: *Magnetic Resonance Imaging of CNS Disease: A Teaching File*, 2nd ed. St. Louis, Mosby, 2002, Case 1083.)

6

Spinal Cord

I. GRAY AND WHITE COMMUNICATING RAMI (Figure 6-1)

A. Gray communicating rami contain unmyelinated postganglionic sympathetic fibers. They are found at all levels of the spinal cord.

B. White communicating rami contain myelinated preganglionic sympathetic fibers. They are found from T-1 to L-3 (the extent of the lateral horn and the intermediolateral cell column).

II. TERMINATION OF THE CONUS MEDULLARIS (see Figure 2-1) occurs in the newborn at the level of the body of the third lumbar vertebra (L-3). In the adult, it occurs at the level of the lower border of the first lumbar vertebra (L-1).

III. LOCATION OF THE MAJOR MOTOR AND SENSORY NUCLEI OF THE SPINAL CORD

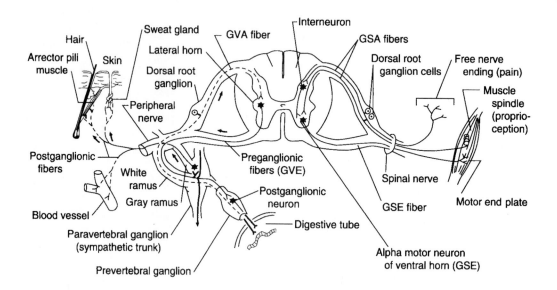

Figure 6-1. The four functional components of the thoracic spinal nerve: general visceral afferent (GVA), general somatic afferent (GSA), general somatic efferent (GSE), and general visceral efferent (GVE). Proprioceptive, cutaneous, and visceral reflex arcs are shown. The muscle stretch (myotatic) reflex includes the muscle spindle, GSA dorsal root ganglion cell, GSE ventral horn motor neuron, and skeletal muscle.

Table 6-1
The Five Most Commonly Tested Muscle Stretch Reflexes

Muscle Stretch Reflex	Cord Segment	Muscle
Ankle jerk	S-1	Gastrocnemius
Knee jerk	L-2–L-4	Quadriceps
Biceps jerk	C-5 and C-6	Biceps
Forearm jerk	C-5–C-6	Brachioradialis
Triceps jerk	C-7 and C-8	Triceps

A. The **ciliospinal center of Budge,** from C-8 to T-2, mediates the sympathetic innervation of the eye.

B. The **intermediolateral cell column,** from C-8 to L-3, mediates the entire sympathetic innervation of the body.

C. The **nucleus dorsalis of Clark,** from C-8 to L-3, gives rise to the dorsal spinocerebellar tract.

D. The **parasympathetic nucleus,** from S-2 to S-4

E. The **spinal accessory nucleus,** from C-1 to C-6

F. The **phrenic nucleus,** from C-3 to C-6

IV. THE CAUDA EQUINA. Motor and sensory roots (L-2 to Co) that are found in the subarachnoid space below the conus medullaris form the cauda equina. They exit the vertebral canal through the lumbar intervertebral and sacral foramina.

V. THE MYOTATIC REFLEX (see Figure 6-1) is a monosynaptic and ipsilateral **muscle stretch reflex (MSR).** Like all reflexes, the myotatic reflex has an afferent and an efferent limb. **Interruption of either limb** results in **areflexia.**

A. The **afferent limb** includes a muscle spindle (receptor) and a dorsal root ganglion neuron and its Ia fiber.

B. The **efferent limb** includes a ventral horn motor neuron that innervates striated muscle (effector).

C. The **four most commonly tested MSRs** are listed in Table 6-1.

7

Tracts of the Spinal Cord

I. INTRODUCTION. Figure 7-1 shows the ascending and descending tracts of the spinal cord. This chapter covers four of the major tracts.

II. DORSAL COLUMN–MEDIAL LEMNISCUS PATHWAY (Figure 7-2; see also Figure 8-1)

   A. Function. The dorsal column—medial lemniscus pathway mediates tactile discrimination, vibration sensation, form recognition, and joint and muscle sensation (conscious proprioception).

   B. Receptors include Pacini's and Meissner's tactile corpuscles, joint receptors, muscle spindles, and Golgi tendon organs.

   C. First-order neurons are located in the dorsal root ganglia at all levels. They project axons to the spinal cord through the medial root entry zone. First-order neurons give rise to:

   1. The gracile fasciculus from the lower extremity

   2. The cuneate fasciculus from the upper extremity

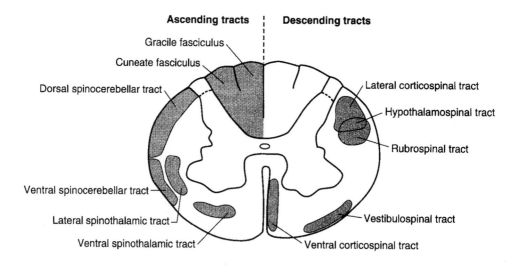

Figure 7-1. The major ascending and descending pathways of the spinal cord. The ascending sensory tracts are shown on the *left,* and the descending motor tracts are shown on the *right.*

Figure 7-2.   The dorsal column–medial lemniscus pathway. Impulses conducted by this pathway mediate discriminatory tactile sense (e.g., touch, vibration, pressure) and kinesthetic sense (e.g., position, movement). The dorsal column system mediates conscious proprioception. (Adapted with permission from Carpenter MB, Sutin J: *Human Neuroanatomy.* Baltimore, Williams & Wilkins, 1983, p. 266.)

     3. The collaterals for spinal reflexes (e.g., myotatic reflex)

     4. The axons that ascend in the dorsal columns and terminate in the gracile and cuneate nuclei of the caudal medulla

  D. **Second-order neurons** are located in the gracile and cuneate nuclei of the caudal medulla. They give rise to axons and internal arcuate fibers that decussate and form a compact fiber bundle (i.e., medial lemniscus). The medial lemniscus ascends through the contralateral brain stem and terminates in the ventral posterolateral (VPL) nucleus of the thalamus.

  E. **Third-order neurons** are located in the VPL nucleus of the thalamus. They project through the posterior limb of the internal capsule to the postcentral gyrus, which is the primary somatosensory cortex (Brodmann's areas 3, 1, and 2).

  F. **Transection of the dorsal column-medial lemniscus tract**

     1. **Above the sensory decussation,** transection results in contralateral loss of the dorsal column modalities.

     2. **In the spinal cord,** transection results in ipsilateral loss of the dorsal column modalities.

III. LATERAL SPINOTHALAMIC TRACT (Figure 7-3; see also Figure 8-1)

  A. **Function.** The lateral spinothalamic tract mediates pain and temperature sensation.

  B. **Receptors** are free nerve endings. The lateral spinothalamic tract receives input from fast- and slow-conducting pain fibers (i.e., A-δ and C, respectively).

  C. **First-order neurons** are found in the dorsal root ganglia at all levels. They project axons to the spinal cord through the dorsolateral tract of Lissauer (lateral root entry zone) to second-order neurons.

  D. **Second-order neurons** are found in the dorsal horn. They give rise to axons that decussate in the **ventral white commissure** and ascend in the contralateral lateral funiculus. Their axons terminate in the VPS nucleus of the thalamus.

  E. **Third-order neurons** are found in the VPL nucleus of the thalamus. They project through the posterior limb of the internal capsule to the primary somatosensory cortex (Brodmann's areas 3, 1, and 2).

  F. **Transection of the lateral spinothalamic tract** results in contralateral loss of pain and temperature below the lesion.

IV. LATERAL CORTICOSPINAL TRACT (Figure 7-4; see also Figure 8-1)

  A. **Function.** The lateral corticospinal tract mediates voluntary skilled motor activity, primarily of the upper limbs. It is not fully myelinated until the end of the second year (Babinski's sign).

  B. **Fiber caliber.** Approximately 90% of the fibers lie between 1 and 4μm, and 4% lie above 20μm (from the giant cells of Betz).

  C. **Origin and termination**

     1. **Origin.** The lateral corticospinal tract arises from layer V of the cerebral cortex from three cortical areas in equal aliquots:

       a. The **premotor cortex** (Brodmann's area 6)

       b. The **primary cortex** (Brodmann's area 4)

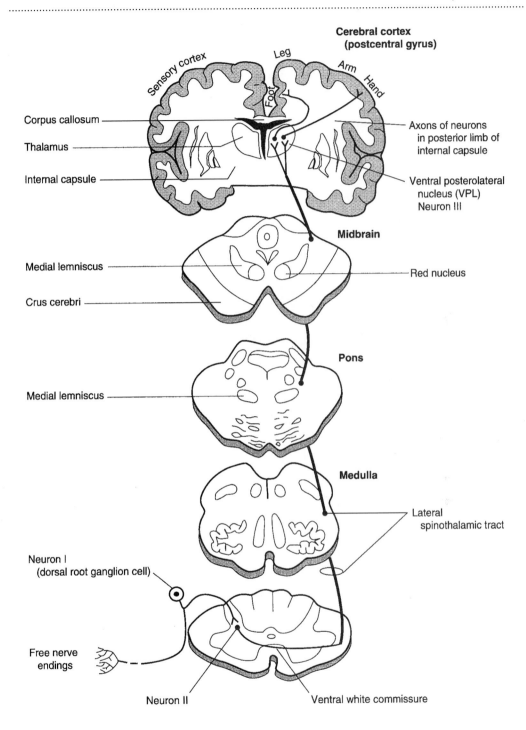

Figure 7-3.   The lateral spinothalamic tract. Impulses conducted by this tract mediate pain and thermal sense. Numerous collaterals are distributed to the brain stem reticular formation. (Reprinted with permission from Carpenter MB, Sutin J: *Human Neuroanatomy.* Baltimore, Williams & Wilkins, 1983, p. 274.)

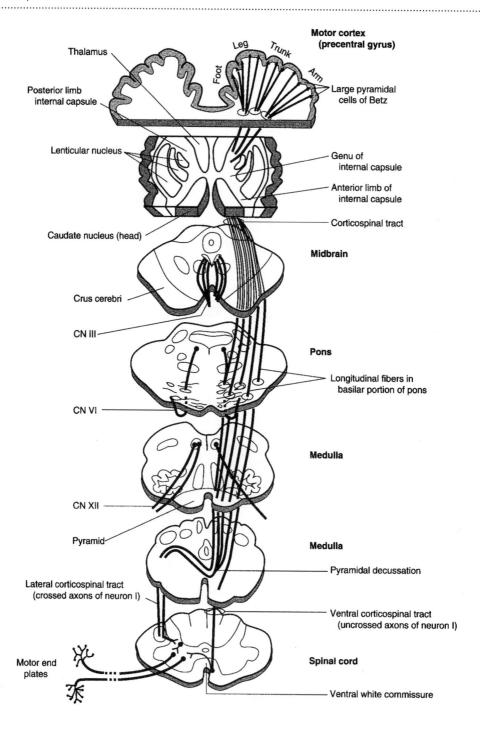

Figure 7-4. The lateral and ventral corticospinal (pyramidal) tracts. These major descending motor pathways mediate volitional motor activity. The cells of origin are located in the premotor, the motor, and the sensory cortices. *CN* = cranial nerve. (Reprinted with permission from Carpenter MB, Sutin J: *Human Neuroanatomy.* Baltimore, Williams & Wilkins, 1983, p. 285.)

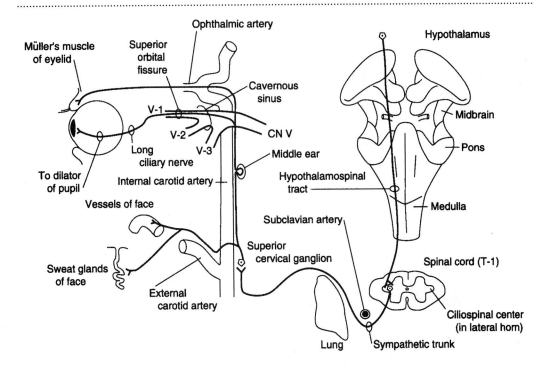

Figure 7-5. The oculosympathetic pathway. Hypothalamic fibers project to the ipsilateral ciliospinal center of the intermediolateral cell column at T-1. The ciliospinal center projects preganglionic sympathetic fibers to the superior cervical ganglion. The superior cervical ganglion projects perivascular postganglionic sympathetic fibers through the tympanic cavity, cavernous sinus, and superior orbital fissure to the dilator muscle of the iris. Interruption of this pathway at any level results in Horner's syndrome. *CN* = cranial nerve.

    c. The **primary sensory cortex** (Brodmann's areas 3, 1, and 2)

    d. Arm, face, and foot areas. The arm and face areas of the motor homunculus arise from the lateral convexity; the foot region of the motor homunculus is found in the paracentral lobule (see Figure 23-2).

  2. Termination. The lateral corticospinal tract terminates contralaterally, through interneurons, on ventral horn motor neurons.

D. Course of the lateral corticospinal tract

  1. Telencephalon. The lateral corticospinal tract runs in the posterior limb of the internal capsule in the telencephalon.

  2. Midbrain. The lateral corticospinal tract runs in the middle three-fifths of the crus cerebri in the midbrain.

  3. Pons. The lateral corticospinal tract runs in the base of the pons.

  4. Medulla. The lateral corticospinal tract runs in the medullary pyramids. Between 85% and 90% of the corticospinal fibers decussate in the pyramidal decussation as the lateral corticospinal tract. The remaining 10% to 15% of the fibers continue as the anterior corticospinal tract.

  5. Spinal cord. The lateral corticospinal tract runs in the dorsal quadrant of the lateral funiculus.

   E. Transection of the lateral corticospinal tract

   1. **Above the motor decussation,** transection results in contralateral spastic paresis and Babinski's sign (upgoing toe).

   2. **In the spinal cord,** transection results in ipsilateral spastic paresis and Babinski's sign.

V. HYPOTHALAMOSPINAL TRACT (Figure 7-5)

   A. **Anatomic location.** The hypothalamospinal tract projects without interruption from the hypothalamus to the ciliospinal center of the intermediolateral cell column at T-1 to T-2. It is found in the spinal cord at T-1 or above in the dorsolateral quadrant of the lateral funiculus. It is also found in the lateral tegmentum of the medulla, pons, and midbrain.

   B. **Clinical features.** Interruption of this tract at any level results in Horner's syndrome (i.e., miosis, ptosis, hemianhidrosis, and apparent enophthalmos). The signs are always ipsilateral.

8

Lesions of the Spinal Cord

I. **DISEASES OF THE MOTOR NEURONS AND CORTICOSPINAL TRACTS** (Figures 8-1 and 8-2)

 A. **Upper motor neuron (UMN) lesions** are caused by transection of the corticospinal tract or destruction of the cortical cells of origin. They result in **spastic paresis** with pyramidal signs (Babinski's sign).

 B. **Lower motor neuron (LMN) lesions** are caused by damage to the motor neurons. They result in **flaccid paralysis,** areflexia, atrophy, fasciculations, and fibrillations. **Poliomyelitis or Werdnig-Hoffman disease** (see Figure 8-2A) results from damage to the motor neurons.

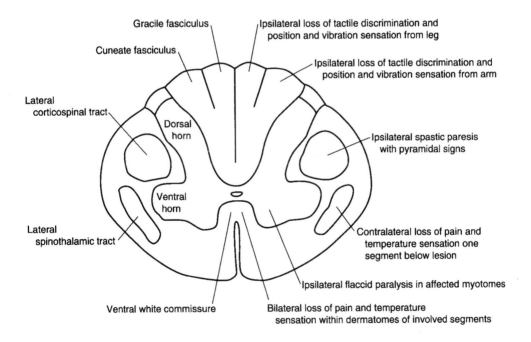

Figure 8-1. Transverse section of the cervical spinal cord. The clinically important ascending and descending pathways are shown on the *left*. Clinical deficits that result from the interruption of these pathways are shown on the *right*. Destructive lesions of the dorsal horns result in anesthesia and areflexia. Destruction of the ventral white commissure interrupts the central transmission of pain and temperature impulses bilaterally through the lateral spinothalamic tracts.

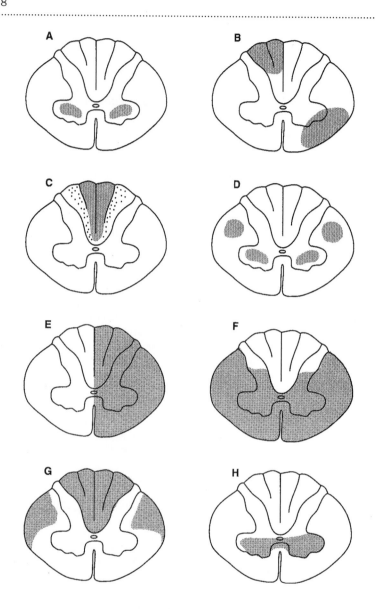

Figure 8-2. Classic lesions of the spinal cord. (A) Poliomyelitis and progressive infantile muscular atrophy (Werdnig-Hoffmann disease). (B) Multiple sclerosis. (C) Dorsal column disease (tabes dorsalis). (D) Amyotrophic lateral sclerosis. (E) Hemisection of the spinal cord (Brown-Séquard syndrome). (F) Complete ventral spinal artery occlusion of the spinal cord. (G) Subacute combined degeneration (vitamin B_{12} neuropathy). (H) Syringomyelia.

 C. Combined UMN and LMN disease. An example of a combined UMN and LMN disease is **amyotrophic lateral sclerosis (ALS, or Lou Gehrig's disease)** [see Figure 8-2D]. ALS is caused by damage to the corticospinal tracts, with pyramidal signs, and by damage to the LMNs, with LMN symptoms. Patients with ALS have no sensory deficits.

II. SENSORY PATHWAY LESIONS. An example of a condition caused by these lesions is **dorsal column disease (tabes dorsalis)** [see Figure 8-2C]. This disease is seen in patients with neurosyphilis. It is characterized by a loss of tactile discrimination and position and vibration sensation. Irritative involvement of the dorsal roots results in pain and paresthesias. Patients have a Romberg sign. (Subject stands with his feet together. When he closes his eyes, he loses his balance. This is a sign of dorsal column ataxia.)

III. COMBINED MOTOR AND SENSORY LESIONS

A. **Spinal cord hemisection (Brown-Séquard syndrome)** [see Figure 8-2E] is caused by damage to the following structures:

  1. The **dorsal columns [gracile (leg) and cuneate (arm) fasciculi]**. Damage results in ipsilateral loss of tactile discrimination and position and vibration sensation.

  2. The **lateral corticospinal tract**. Damage results in ipsilateral spastic paresis with pyramidal signs below the lesion.

  3. The **lateral spinothalamic tract**. Damage results in contralateral loss of pain and temperature sensation one segment below the lesion.

  4. The **hypothalamospinal tract at T-1 and above**. Damage results in ipsilateral Horner's syndrome (i.e., miosis, ptosis, hemianhidrosis, and apparent enophthalmos).

  5. The **ventral (anterior) horn**. Damage results in ipsilateral flaccid paralysis of innervated muscles.

B. **Ventral spinal artery occlusion** (see Figure 8-2F) causes infarction of the anterior two-thirds of the spinal cord but spares the dorsal columns and horns. It results in damage to the following structures:

  1. The **lateral corticospinal tracts**. Damage results in bilateral spastic paresis with pyramidal signs below the lesion.

  2. The **lateral spinothalamic tracts**. Damage results in bilateral loss of pain and temperature sensation below the lesion.

  3. The **hypothalamospinal tract at T-2 and above**. Damage results in bilateral Horner's syndrome.

  4. The **ventral (anterior) horns**. Damage results in bilateral flaccid paralysis of the innervated muscles.

  5. The **corticospinal tracts to the sacral parasympathetic centers at S-2 to S-4**. Damage results in bilateral damage and loss of voluntary bladder and bowel control.

C. **Subacute combined degeneration (vitamin B$_{12}$ neuropathy)** [see Figure 8-2G] is caused by pernicious (megaloblastic) anemia. It results from damage to the following structures:

  1. The **dorsal columns (gracile and cuneate fasciculi)**. Damage results in bilateral loss of tactile discrimination and position and vibration sensation.

  2. The **lateral corticospinal tracts**. Damage results in bilateral spastic paresis with pyramidal signs.

  3. The **spinocerebellar tracts**. Damage results in bilateral arm and leg dystaxia.

D. **Syringomyelia** (see Figure 8-2H) is a central cavitation of the cervical cord of unknown etiology. It results in damage to the following structures:

1. The **ventral white commissure.** Damage to decussating lateral spinothalamic axons causes bilateral loss of pain and temperature sensation.

2. The **ventral horns.** LMN lesions result in flaccid paralysis of the intrinsic muscles of the hands.

E. Friedreich's ataxia has the same spinal cord pathology and symptoms as subacute combined degeneration.

F. Multiple sclerosis (see Figure 8-2B). Plaques primarily involve the white matter of the cervical segments of the spinal cord. The lesions are random and asymmetric.

IV. PERIPHERAL NERVOUS SYSTEM (PNS) LESIONS. An example of a PNS lesion is **Guillain-Barré syndrome** (acute idiopathic polyneuritis, or postinfectious polyneuritis). It primarily affects the motor fibers of the ventral roots and peripheral nerves, and it produces LMN symptoms (i.e., muscle weakness, ascending flaccid paralysis, and areflexia.) Guillain-Barré syndrome has the following features:

A. It is characterized by demyelination and edema.

B. Upper cervical root (C4) involvement and respiratory paralysis are common.

C. Caudal cranial nerve involvement with facial diplegia is present in 50% of cases.

D. Elevated protein levels may cause papilledema.

E. To a lesser degree, sensory fibers are affected, resulting in paresthesias.

F. The protein level in the cerebrospinal fluid is elevated, but without pleocytosis **(albuminocytologic dissociation).**

V. INTERVERTEBRAL DISK HERNIATION is seen at the L-4 to L-5 or L-5 to S-1 interspace in 90% of cases. It appears at the C-5 to C-6 or C-6 to C-7 interspace in 10% of cases.

A. Intervertebral disk herniation consists of prolapse, or herniation, of the **nucleus pulposus through the defective anulus fibrosus and into the vertebral canal.**

B. The nucleus pulposus **impinges on the spinal roots,** resulting in spinal root symptoms (i.e., paresthesias, pain, sensory loss, hyporeflexia, and muscle weakness).

VI. CAUDA EQUINA SYNDROME (SPINAL ROOTS L3 TO CO) results usually from a nerve root tumor, an ependymoma, a dermoid tumor, or from a lipoma of the terminal cord. Is characterized by:

A. Severe radicular unilateral pain

B. Sensory distribution in unilateral **saddle-shaped** area

C. Unilateral muscle atrophy and absent quadriceps (L3) and ankle jerks (S1)

D. Incontinence and sexual functions are not marked

E. Onset gradual and unilateral

VII. CONUS MEDULLARIS SYNDROME (CORD SEGMENTS S3 TO CO) usually results from an intramedullary tumor (e.g., ependymoma). Is characterized by:

A. Pain usually bilateral and not severe

B. Sensory distribution in bilateral **saddle-shaped** area

C. Muscle changes not marked; quadriceps and ankle reflexes normal

D. Incontinence and sexual functions severly impaired

E. Onset sudden and bilateral

9

Brain Stem

I. **OVERVIEW.** The brain stem includes the **medulla, pons,** and **midbrain.** It extends from the pyramidal decussation to the posterior commissure. The brain stem receives its blood supply from the vertebrobasilar system. It contains cranial nerves (CN) III to XII (except the spinal part of CN XI). Figures 9-1 and 9-2 show its surface anatomy.

II. **CROSS-SECTION THROUGH THE MEDULLA** (Figure 9-3)

A. Medial structures

1. The **hypoglossal nucleus of CN XII**

2. The **medial lemniscus,** which contains crossed fibers from the gracile and cuneate nuclei

3. The **pyramid** (corticospinal tracts)

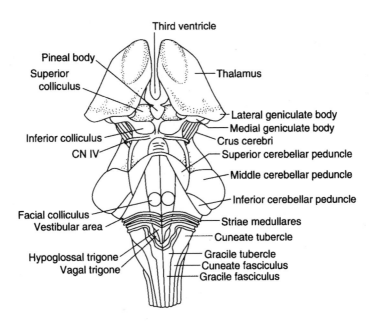

Figure 9-1. The dorsal surface of the brain stem. The three cerebellar peduncles have been removed to expose the rhomboid fossa. The trochlear nerve is the only nerve to exit the brain stem from the dorsal surface. The facial colliculus surmounts the genu of the facial nerve and the abducent nucleus. *CN* = cranial nerve.

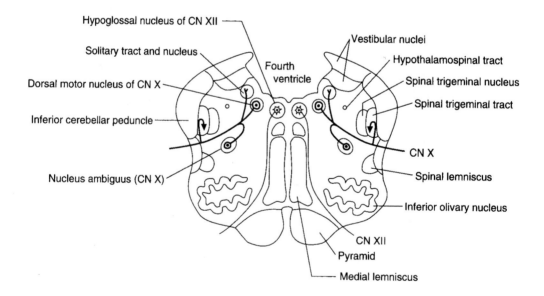

Figure 9-2.   The ventral surface of the brain stem and the attached cranial nerves (CN).

Figure 9-3.   Transverse section of the medulla at the midolivary level. The vagal nerve [cranial nerve (CN) X], hypoglossal nerve (CN XII), and vestibular nerve (CN VIII) are prominent in this section. The nucleus ambiguus gives rise to special visceral efferent fibers to CN IX, X, and XI.

B. Lateral structures

    1. The **nucleus ambiguus (CN IX, X, and XI)**

    2. The **vestibular nuclei (CN VIII)**

    3. The **inferior cerebellar peduncle,** which contains the dorsal spinocerebellar, cuneocerebellar, and olivocerebellar tracts

    4. The **lateral spinothalamic tract** (spinal lemniscus)

    5. The **spinal trigeminal nucleus** and **tract of CN V**

III. CROSS-SECTION THROUGH THE PONS (Figure 9-4). The pons has a dorsal tegmentum and a ventral base.

A. Medial structures

    1. Medial longitudinal fasciculus

    2. Abducent nucleus of CN VI (underlies facial colliculus)

    3. Genu (internal) of CN VII (underlies facial nerve) [facial colliculus]

    4. Abducent fibers of CN VI

    5. Medial lemniscus

    6. Corticospinal tract (in the base of the pons)

B. Lateral structures

    1. Facial nucleus (CN VII)

    2. Facial (intraaxial) nerve fibers

    3. Spinal trigeminal nucleus and tract (CN V)

    4. Lateral spinothalamic tract (spinal lemniscus)

    5. Vestibular nuclei of CN VIII

    6. Cochlear nuclei of CN VIII

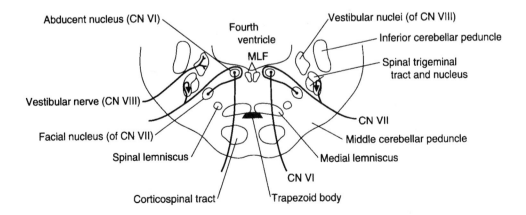

Figure 9-4. Transverse section of the pons at the level of the abducent nucleus of cranial nerve (CN) VI and the facial nucleus of CN VII. *MLF* = medial longitudinal fasciculus.

Figure 9-5.   Transverse section of the midbrain at the level of the superior colliculus, oculomotor nucleus of cranial nerve (CN) III, and red nucleus. *MLF* = medial longitudinal fasciculus.

IV. CROSS-SECTION THROUGH THE ROSTRAL MIDBRAIN (Figure 9-5). The midbrain has a dorsal tectum, an intermediate tegmentum, and a base. The aqueduct lies between the tectum and the tegmentum.

   A. **Dorsal structures** include the **superior colliculi**.

   B. Tegmentum

   1. Oculomotor nucleus (CN III)

   2. Medial longitudinal fasciculus

   3. Red nucleus

   4. Substantia nigra

   5. Dentatothalamic tract (crossed)

   6. Medial lemniscus

   7. Lateral spinothalamic tract (in the spinal lemniscus)

   C. **Crus cerebri** (basis pedunculi cerebri, or cerebral peduncle). The **corticospinal tract** lies in the middle three-fifths of the crus cerebri.

V. CORTICOBULBAR FIBERS (see also Figure 13-4) project bilaterally to all motor cranial nerve nuclei except the facial nucleus. The division of the facial nerve nucleus that innervates the **upper face** (the orbicularis oculi muscle and above) **receives bilateral corticobulbar input.** The division of the facial nerve nucleus that innervates the **lower face** **receives** only **contralateral corticobulbar input.**

10
Trigeminal System

I. OVERVIEW. The trigeminal system provides **sensory innervation to the face, oral cavity, and supratentorial dura** through general somatic afferent (GSA) fibers. It also **innervates the muscles of mastication** through special visceral efferent (SVE) fibers.

II. THE TRIGEMINAL GANGLION (semilunar or gasserian) contains pseudounipolar ganglion cells. It has three divisions:

A. The **ophthalmic nerve [cranial nerve (CN) V-1]** lies in the wall of the cavernous sinus. It enters the orbit through the superior orbital fissure and innervates the forehead, dorsum of the nose, upper eyelid, orbit (cornea and conjunctiva), and cranial dura. The ophthalmic nerve mediates the afferent limb of the corneal reflex.

B. The **maxillary nerve (CN V-2)** lies in the wall of the cavernous sinus and innervates the upper lip and cheek, lower eyelid, anterior portion of the temple, oral mucosa of the upper mouth, nose, pharynx, gums, teeth and palate of the upper jaw, and cranial dura. It exits the skull through the foramen rotundum.

C. The **mandibular nerve (CN V-3)** exits the skull through the foramen ovale. Its **sensory (GSA) component** innervates the lower lip and chin, posterior portion of the temple, external auditory meatus, and tympanic membrane, external ear, teeth of the lower jaw, oral mucosa of the cheeks and floor of the mouth, anterior two-thirds of the tongue, temporomandibular joint, and cranial dura.

D. The **motor (SVE) component** of CN V accompanies the mandibular nerve (CN V-3) through the foramen ovale. It innervates the muscles of mastication, mylohyoid, anterior belly of the digastric, and tensores tympani and veli palatini. It innervates the muscles that move the jaw, the lateral and medial pterygoids (Figure 10-1).

III. TRIGEMINOTHALAMIC PATHWAYS (Figure 10-2)

A. The **ventral trigeminothalamic tract** mediates pain and temperature sensation from the face and oral cavity.

    1. First-order neurons are located in the trigeminal (gasserian) ganglion. They give rise to axons that descend in the spinal trigeminal tract and synapse with second-order neurons in the spinal trigeminal nucleus.

    2. Second-order neurons are located in the spinal trigeminal nucleus. They give rise to decussating axons that terminate in the contralateral ventral posteromedial (VPM) nucleus of the thalamus.

    3. Third-order neurons are located in the VPM nucleus of the thalamus. They

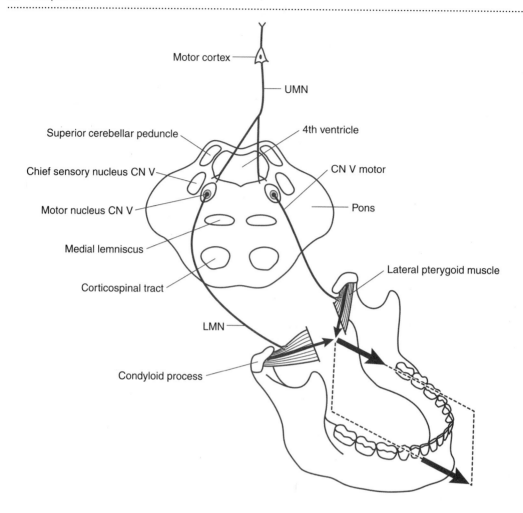

Figure 10-1. Function and innervation of the lateral pterygoid muscles (LPMs). The LPM receives its innervation from the motor nucleus of the trigeminal nerve found in the rostral pons. Bilateral innervation of the LPMs results in protrusion of the tip of the mandible in the midline. The LPMs also open the jaw. Denervation of one LPM results in deviation of the mandible to the ipsilateral or weak side. The trigeminal motor nucleus receives bilateral corticobulbar input. CN = cranial nerve; LMN = lower motor neuron; UMN = upper motor neuron.

project through the posterior limb of the internal capsule to the face area of the somatosensory cortex (Brodmann's areas 3, 1, and 2).

   B. The **dorsal trigeminothalamic tract** mediates tactile discrimination and pressure sensation from the face and oral cavity. It receives input from Meissner's and Pacini's corpuscles.

   1. First-order neurons are located in the trigeminal (gasserian) ganglion. They synapse in the principal sensory nucleus of CN V.

   2. Second-order neurons are located in the principal sensory nucleus of CN V. They project to the ipsilateral VPM nucleus of the thalamus.

Figure 10-2. The ventral (pain and temperature) and dorsal (discriminative touch) trigeminothalamic pathways. CN = cranial nerve.

  3. Third-order neurons are located in the VPM nucleus of the thalamus. They project through the posterior limb of the internal capsule to the face area of the somatosensory cortex (Brodmann's areas 3, 1, and 2).

IV. TRIGEMINAL REFLEXES

  A. Introduction (Table 10-1)

  1. The **corneal reflex** is a consensual disynaptic reflex.

Table 10-1
The Trigeminal Reflexes

Reflex	Afferent Limb	Efferent Limb
Corneal reflex	Ophthalmic nerve (CN V-1)	Facial nerve (CN VII)
Jaw jerk	Mandibular nerve (CN V-3)*	Mandibular nerve (CN V-3)
Tearing (lacrimal) reflex	Ophthalmic nerve (CN V-1)	Facial nerve (CN VII)
Oculocardiac reflex	Ophthalmic nerve (CN V-1)	Vagal nerve (CN X)

*The cell bodies are found in the mesencephalic nucleus of CN V.
CN = cranial nerve.

  2. The **jaw jerk reflex** is a monosynaptic myotatic reflex (Figure 10-3).

  3. The **tearing (lacrimal) reflex**

  4. The **oculocardiac reflex** occurs when pressure on the globe results in **bradycardia**.

B. Clinical correlation. Trigeminal neuralgia (tic douloureux) is characterized by recurrent paroxysms of sharp, stabbing pain in one or more branches of the trigeminal nerve on one side of the face. It usually occurs in people older than 50 years of age, and it is more common in women than in men. **Carbamazepine** is the drug of choice for idiopathic trigeminal neuralgia.

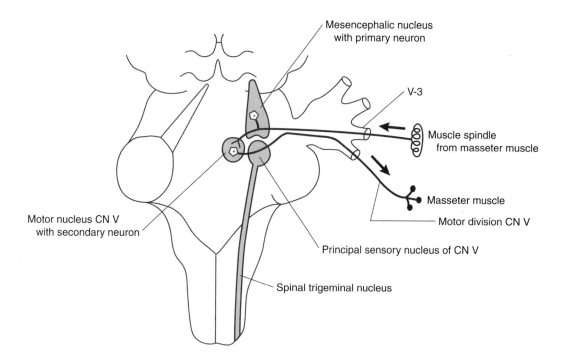

Figure 10-3. The jaw jerk (masseter) reflex. The afferent limb is V-3, and the efferent limb is the motor root that accompanies V-3. First-order sensory neurons are located in the mesencephalic nucleus. The jaw jerk reflex, like all muscle stretch reflexes, is a monosynaptic myotactic reflex. Hyperreflexia indicates an upper motor neuron lesion. CN = cranial nerve.

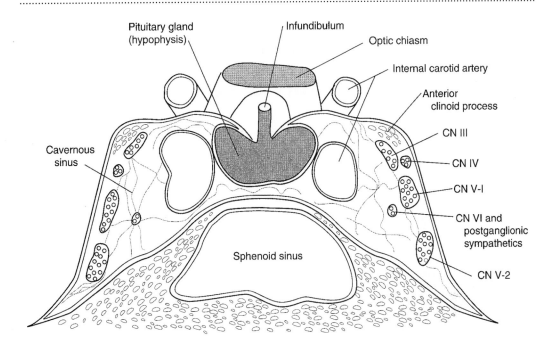

Figure 10-4.   The contents of the cavernous sinus. The wall of the cavernous sinus contains the ophthalmic cranial nerve (CN) V-1 and maxillary (CN V-2) divisions of the trigeminal nerve (CN V) and the trochlear (CN IV) and oculomotor (CN III) nerves. The siphon of the internal carotid artery and the abducent nerve (CN VI), along with postganglionic sympathetic fibers, lies within the cavernous sinus.

V. THE CAVERNOUS SINUS (Figure 10-4) contains the following structures:

   A. **Internal carotid artery** (siphon)

   B. **CN III, IV, V-1, V-2,** and **VI**

   C. **Postganglionic sympathetic fibers** en route to the orbit

11

Auditory System

I. OVERVIEW. The auditory system is an exteroceptive special somatic afferent system that can detect sound frequencies from 20 Hz to 20,000 Hz. It is derived from the **otic vesicle,** which is a derivative of the **otic placode,** a thickening of the **surface ectoderm.**

II. THE AUDITORY PATHWAY (Figure 11-1) consists of the following structures.

    A. The **hair cells of the organ of Corti** are innervated by the peripheral processes of bipolar cells of the spiral ganglion. They are stimulated by vibrations of the basilar membrane.

        1. Inner hair cells are the chief sensory elements; they synapse with dendrites of myelinated neurons whose axons comprise 90% of the cochlear nerve.

        2. Outer hair cells synapse with dendrites of unmyelinated neurons whose axons comprise 10% of the cochlear nerve. The OHCs reduce the threshold of the IHCs.

    B. The **bipolar cells of the spiral (cochlear) ganglion** project peripherally to the hair cells of the organ of Corti. They project centrally as the cochlear nerve to the cochlear nuclei.

    C. The **cochlear nerve [cranial nerve (CN) VIII]** extends from the spiral ganglion to the cerebellopontine angle, where it enters the brain stem.

    D. The **cochlear nuclei** receive input from the cochlear nerve. They project contralaterally to the superior olivary nucleus and lateral lemniscus.

    E. The **superior olivary nucleus,** which plays a role in sound localization, receives input from the cochlear nuclei. It projects to the lateral lemniscus.

    F. The **trapezoid body** is located in the pons. It contains decussating fibers from the ventral cochlear nuclei.

    G. The **lateral lemniscus** receives input from the contralateral cochlear nuclei and superior olivary nuclei.

    H. The **nucleus of inferior colliculus** receives input from the lateral lemniscus. It projects through the brachium of the inferior colliculus to the medial geniculate body.

    I. The **medial geniculate body** receives input from the nucleus of inferior colliculus. It projects through the internal capsule as the auditory radiation to the primary auditory cortex, the transverse temporal gyri of Heschl.

    J. The **transverse temporal gyri of Heschl** contain the primary auditory cortex (Brodmann's areas 41 and 42). The gyri are located in the depths of the lateral sulcus.

III. HEARING DEFECTS

    A. Conduction deafness is caused by interruption of the passage of sound waves through the external or middle ear. It may be caused by **obstruction** (e.g., wax), **otosclerosis,** or **otitis media.**

Figure 11-1.   Peripheral and central connections of the auditory system. This system arises from the hair cells of the organ of Corti and terminates in the transverse temporal gyri of Heschl of the superior temporal gyrus. It is characterized by the bilaterality of projections and the tonotopic localization of pitch at all levels. For example, high pitch (20,000 Hz) is localized at the base of the cochlea and in the posteromedial part of the transverse temporal gyri. CN = cranial nerve.

   B. Nerve deafness (sensorineural, or perceptive, deafness) is caused by disease of the cochlea, cochlear nerve (acoustic neuroma), or central auditory connections. It is usually caused by **presbycusis** that results from degenerative disease of the organ of Corti in the first few millimeters of the basal coil of the cochlea (high-frequency loss of 4000–8000 Hz).

IV. AUDITORY TESTS
   A. Tuning fork tests (Table 11-1)

Table 11-1
Tuning Fork Test Results

Otologic Finding	Weber Test	Rinne Test
Conduction deafness (left ear)	Lateralizes to left ear	BC >AC on left AC >BC on right
Conduction deafness (right ear)	Lateralizes to right ear	BC >AC on right AC >BC on left
Nerve deafness (left ear)	Lateralizes to right ear	AC >BC, both ears
Nerve deafness (right ear)	Lateralizes to left ear	AC >BC, both ears
Normal ears	No laterlization	AC >BC, both ears

Conduction deafness = middle ear deafness (e.g., otosclerosis, otitis media); nerve deafness = sensorineural deafness (e.g., presbycusis; AC = air conduction: BC = bone conduction.

1. **Weber's test** is performed by placing a vibrating tuning fork on the vertex of the skull. Normally, a patient hears equally on both sides.

   a. A patient who has **unilateral conduction deafness** hears the vibration more loudly in the affected ear.

   b. A patient who has **unilateral partial nerve deafness** hears the vibration more loudly in the normal ear.

2. **The Rinne test compares air and bone conduction. It is performed by placing a vibrating tuning fork on the mastoid process until the vibration is no longer heard; then the fork is held in front of the ear. Normally, a patient hears the vibration in the air after bone conduction is gone.**

   a. A patient who has **unilateral conduction deafness** does not hear the vibration in the air after bone conduction is gone.

   b. A patient who has **unilateral partial nerve deafness** hears the vibration in the air after bone conduction is gone.

B. Brain stem auditory evoked potentials (BAEPs)

   1. **Testing method.** Clicks are presented to one ear, then to the other. Scalp electrodes and a computer generate a series of seven waves. The waves are associated with specific areas of the auditory pathway.

   2. **Diagnostic value.** This method is valuable for diagnosing brain stem lesions **(multiple sclerosis)** and posterior fossa tumors **(acoustic neuromas).** It is also useful for assessing hearing in infants. Approximately 50% of patients with multiple sclerosis have abnormal BAEPs.

12

Vestibular System

I. OVERVIEW. Like the auditory system, the vestibular system is derived from the **otic vesicle.** The otic vesicle is a derivative of the **otic placode,** which is a thickening of the **surface ectoderm.** This system maintains **posture** and **equilibrium** and coordinates **head and eye movements.**

II. THE LABYRINTH

   A. Kinetic labyrinth

      1. **Three semicircular ducts** lie within the three semicircular canals (i.e., superior, lateral, and posterior).

      2. These ducts **respond to angular acceleration and deceleration of the head.**

         a. They contain **hair cells** in the crista ampullaris. The hair cells **respond to endolymph flow.**

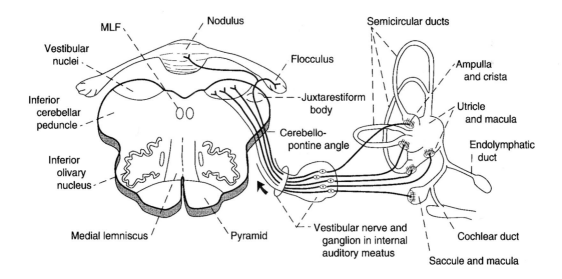

Figure 12-1. Peripheral connections of the vestibular system. The hair cells of the cristae ampullares and the maculae of the utricle and saccule project, through the vestibular nerve, to the vestibular nuclei of the medulla and pons and the flocculonodular lobe of the cerebellum (vestibulocerebellum). *MLF* = medial longitudinal fasciculus.

   b. Endolymph flow toward the ampulla (ampullopetal) or utricle (utriculopetal) is a stronger stimulus than is endolymph flow in the opposite direction.

B. Static labyrinth

   1. The **utricle** and **saccule** respond to the position of the head with respect to **linear acceleration** and the pull of **gravity.**

   2. The utricle and saccule contain **hair cells** whose cilia are embedded in the otolithic membrane. When hair cells are bent toward the longest cilium (kinocilium), the frequency of sensory discharge increases.

III. THE VESTIBULAR PATHWAYS (Figures 12-1 and 12-2) consist of the following structures.

   A. **Hair cells of the semicircular ducts, saccule, and utricle** are innervated by peripheral processes of **bipolar cells** of the vestibular ganglion.

Figure 12-2. The major central connections of the vestibular system. Vestibular nuclei project through the ascending medial longitudinal fasciculi (*MLF*) to the ocular motor nuclei and subserve vestibulo-ocular reflexes. Vestibular nuclei also project through the descending MLF and lateral vestibulospinal tracts to the ventral horn motor neurons of the spinal cord and mediate postural reflexes. *CN* = cranial nerve.

B. The **vestibular ganglion** is located in the fundus of the internal auditory meatus.

   1. Bipolar neurons project through their peripheral processes to the hair cells.

   2. Bipolar neurons project their central processes as the vestibular nerve [cranial nerve (CN) VIII] to the vestibular nuclei and to the flocculonodular lobe of the cerebellum.

C. Vestibular nuclei

   1. These nuclei receive input from:

     a. The semicircular ducts, saccule, and utricle

     b. The flocculonodular lobe of the cerebellum

   2. The nuclei project fibers to:

     a. The flocculonodular lobe of the cerebellum

     b. CN III, IV, and VI through the medial longitudinal fasciculus (MLF)

     c. The spinal cord through the lateral vestibulospinal tract

     d. The ventral posteroinferior and posterolateral nuclei of the thalamus, both of which project to the postcentral gyrus

IV. VESTIBULO-OCULAR REFLEXES are mediated by the vestibular nuclei, MLF, ocular motor nuclei, and CN III, IV, and VI.

A. Vestibular (horizontal) nystagmus

   1. The **fast phase** of nystagmus is in the **direction of rotation.**

   2. The **slow phase** of nystagmus is in the **opposite direction.**

B. Postrotatory (horizontal) nystagmus

   1. The **fast phase** of nystagmus is in the **opposite direction of rotation.**

   2. The **slow phase** of nystagmus is in the **direction of rotation.**

   3. The patient past-points and falls in the direction of previous rotation.

C. Caloric nystagmus (stimulation of horizontal ducts) in normal subjects

   1. Cold water irrigation of the external auditory meatus results in nystagmus to the opposite side.

   2. Warm water irrigation of the external auditory meatus results in nystagmus to the same side.

Normal conscious subject   Brain stem intact   MLF (bilateral) lesion   Low brain stem lesion

Figure 12-3. Cold caloric responses in the unconscious patient. When the brain stem is intact, the eyes deviate toward the irrigated side; with bilateral transection of the medial longitudinal fasciculi (*MLF*), the eye deviates to the abducted side. Destruction of the caudal brain stem results in no deviation of the eyes. *Double-headed arrows* indicate nystagmus; *single-headed arrows* indicate deviation of the eyes to one side.

3. Remember the mnemonic COWS: Cold Opposite, Warm Same.

D. Test results in **unconscious subjects** (Figure 12-3)

1. No nystagmus is seen.

2. When the brain stem is intact, there is deviation of the eyes to the side of the cold irrigation.

3. With bilateral MLF transection, there is deviation of the abducting eye to the side of the cold irrigation.

4. With lower brain stem damage to the vestibular nuclei, there is no deviation of the eyes.

13

Cranial Nerves

I. THE OLFACTORY NERVE, the first cranial nerve **(CN I)** [Figure 13-1], mediates olfaction **(smell).** It is the only sensory system that has no precortical relay in the thalamus. The olfactory nerve is a special visceral afferent (SVA) nerve. It consists of unmyelinated axons of bipolar neurons that are located in the nasal mucosa, the olfactory epithelium. It enters the skull through the cribriform plate of the ethmoid bone (see appendix).

A. Olfactory pathway

    1. Olfactory receptor cells are first-order neurons that project to the mitral cells of the olfactory bulb.

    2. Mitral cells are the principal cells of the olfactory bulb. They are excitatory and glutaminergic. They project through the **olfactory tract** and **lateral olfactory stria** to the primary olfactory cortex and amygdala.

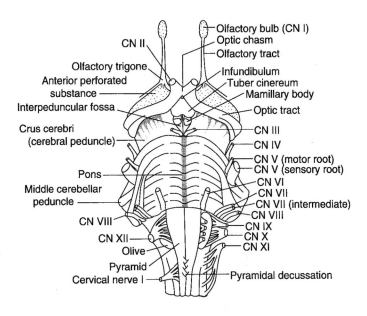

Figure 13-1. The base of the brain with attached cranial nerves (CN). (Reprinted with permission from Truex RC, Kellner CE: *Detailed Atlas of the Head and Neck*. New York, Oxford University Press, 1958, p. 34.)

3. The primary olfactory cortex (Brodmann's area 34) consists of the piriform cortex that overlies the uncus.

B. Lesions of the olfactory pathway result from trauma (e.g., skull fracture) and, often, from olfactory groove meningiomas. These lesions cause **ipsilateral anosmia** (localizing value). Lesions that involve the parahippocampal uncus may cause olfactory hallucinations [uncinate fits (seizures) with déjà vu].

C. Foster Kennedy syndrome (FKS) consists of ipsilateral anosmia, ipsilateral optic atrophy, and contralateral papilledema. It is usually caused by an anterior fossa meningioma.

II. THE OPTIC NERVE (CN II) is a special somatic afferent **(SSA)** nerve that subserves vision and pupillary light reflexes (afferent limb) [see Chapter 19]. It is **not a true peripheral nerve,** but is a tract of the diencephalon. A transected optic nerve cannot regenerate.

III. THE OCULOMOTOR NERVE (CN III) is a general somatic efferent (GSE), general visceral efferent (GVE) nerve.

A. General characteristics. The oculomotor nerve **moves** the **eye, constricts** the **pupil, accommodates,** and **converges.** It exits the brain stem from the interpeduncular fossa of the midbrain, passes through the cavernous sinus, and enters the orbit through the superior orbital fissure.

1. The **GSE component** arises from the oculomotor nucleus of the rostral midbrain. It innervates four extraocular muscles and the levator palpebrae muscle. (Remember the mnemonic **SIN: superior** muscles are **in**torters of the globe.)

a. The **medial rectus muscle** adducts the eye. With its opposite partner, it converges the eyes.

b. The **superior rectus muscle** elevates, intorts, and adducts the eye.

c. The **inferior rectus muscle** depresses, extorts, and adducts the eye.

d. The **inferior oblique muscle** elevates, extorts, and abducts the eye.

e. The **levator palpebrae muscle** elevates the upper eyelid.

2. The **GVE component** consists of preganglionic parasympathetic fibers.

a. The **Edinger-Westphal nucleus** projects preganglionic parasympathetic fibers to the ciliary ganglion of the orbit through CN III.

b. The **ciliary ganglion** projects postganglionic parasympathetic fibers to the sphincter muscle of the iris (miosis) and the ciliary muscle (accommodation).

B. Clinical correlation

1. Oculomotor paralysis (palsy) is seen with transtentorial herniation (e.g., tumor, subdural or epidural hematoma).

a. Denervation of the **levator palpebrae muscle** causes **ptosis** (i.e., drooping of the upper eyelid).

b. Denervation of the **extraocular muscles** causes the affected eye to look "down and out" as a result of the unopposed action of the lateral rectus and superior oblique muscles. The superior oblique and lateral rectus muscles are innervated by CN IV and CN VI, respectively. Oculomotor palsy results in **diplopia** (double vision) when the patient looks in the direction of the paretic muscle.

c. Interruption of parasympathetic innervation (internal ophthalmoplegia) results in a **dilated, fixed pupil** and **paralysis of accommodation** (cycloplegia).

2. Other conditions associated with CN III impairment

a. Transtentorial (uncal) herniation. Increased supratentorial pressure (e.g., from a tumor) forces the hippocampal uncus through the tentorial notch and compresses or stretches the oculomotor nerve.

(1) Pupilloconstrictor fibers are affected first, resulting in a **dilated, fixed pupil.**

(2) Somatic efferent fibers are affected later, resulting in **external strabismus** (exotropia).

b. Aneurysms of the carotid and posterior communicating arteries often compress CN III within the cavernous sinus or interpeduncular cistern. They usually affect the peripheral pupilloconstrictor fibers first (e.g., uncal herniation).

c. Diabetes mellitus (diabetic oculomotor palsy) often affects the oculomotor nerve. It damages the central fibers and spares the pupilloconstrictor fibers.

IV. THE TROCHLEAR NERVE (CN IV) is a GSE nerve.

A. General characteristics. The trochlear nerve is a pure motor nerve that innervates the superior oblique muscle. This muscle depresses, intorts, and abducts the eye. (See Figure 17-4G.)

1. It **arises from** the contralateral trochlear nucleus of the caudal midbrain.

2. It **decussates** beneath the superior medullary velum of the midbrain and exits the brain stem on its dorsal surface, caudal to the inferior colliculus.

3. It **encircles the midbrain** within the subarachnoid space, passes through the cavernous sinus, and enters the orbit through the superior orbital fissure.

B. Clinical correlation. CN IV paralysis results in the following conditions:

1. Extorsion of the eye and weakness of downward gaze

2. Vertical diplopia, which increases when looking down

3. Head tilting to compensate for extorsion (may be misdiagnosed as idiopathic torticollis)

4. Head trauma. Because of its course around the midbrain, the trochlear nerve is particularly vulnerable to head trauma. The trochlear decussation underlies the superior medullary velum. Trauma at this site often results in bilateral fourth-nerve palsies. Pressure against the free border of the tentorium (herniation) may injure the nerve [Figure 13-2].

V. THE TRIGEMINAL NERVE (CN V) is a special visceral efferent (SVE), general somatic afferent (GSA) nerve (see Chapter 10) [Figure 13-3].

A. General characteristics. The trigeminal nerve is the nerve of pharyngeal (brachial) arch 1 (mandibular). It has three divisions: ophthalmic (CN V-1), maxillary (CN V-2), and mandibular (CN V-3) [see Chapter 10].

1. The **SVE component** arises from the motor trigeminal nucleus that is found in the lateral midpontine tegmentum. It **innervates** the **muscles of mastication** (i.e.,

A   **B**

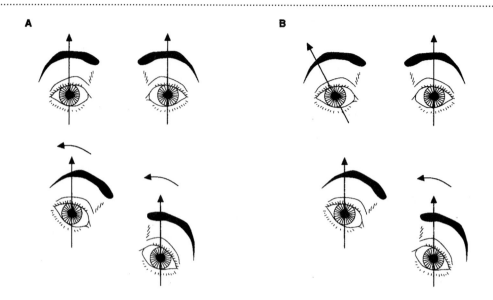

Figure 13-2.   Paralysis of the right superior oblique muscle. (A) A pair of eyes with normal extorsion and intorsion movements. Tilting the chin to the right side results in compensatory intorsion of the left eye and extorsion of the right eye. (B) Paralysis of the right superior oblique muscle results in extorsion of the right eye, causing diplopia. Tilting the chin to the right side results in compensatory intorsion of the left eye, thus permitting binocular alignment. (Reprinted with permission from Fix JD: *BRS Neuroanatomy*, 3rd ed. Baltimore, Williams & Wilkins, 1996, p. 220.)

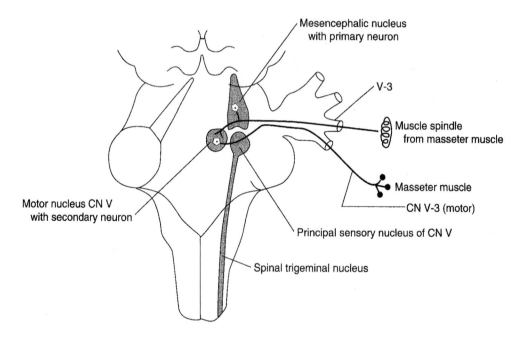

Figure 13-3.   Jaw jerk (masseter reflex) pathway showing two neurons. Note the first-order (sensory) neuron is found in the mesencephalic nucleus of the pons and midbrain, not in the trigeminal ganglion. (Reprinted with permission from Fix JD: *BRS Neuroanatomy*, 3rd ed. Baltimore, Williams & Wilkins, 1996, p. 220.)

temporalis, masseter, lateral, and medial pterygoids), the tensores tympani and veli palatini, the myelohyoid muscle, and the anterior belly of the digastric muscle.

2. The **GSA component** provides **sensory innervation to the face,** mucous membranes of the nasal and oral cavities and frontal sinus, hard palate, and deep structures of the head (proprioception from muscles and the temporomandibular joint). It innervates the dura of the anterior and middle cranial fossae (supratentorial dura).

B. Clinical correlation. Lesions result in the following neurologic deficits:

1. **Loss of general sensation (hemianesthesia)** from the face and mucous membranes of the oral and nasal cavities

2. **Loss of the corneal reflex** (afferent limb, CN V-1) [Figure 13-4]

3. **Flaccid paralysis** of the muscles of mastication

4. **Deviation of the jaw to the weak side** as a result of the unopposed action of the opposite lateral pterygoid muscle

5. **Paralysis of the tensor tympani muscle,** which leads to hypoacusis (partial deafness to low-pitched sounds)

6. **Trigeminal neuralgia** (tic douloureux), which is characterized by recurrent paroxysms of sharp, stabbing pain in one or more branches of the nerve (see Chapter 10)

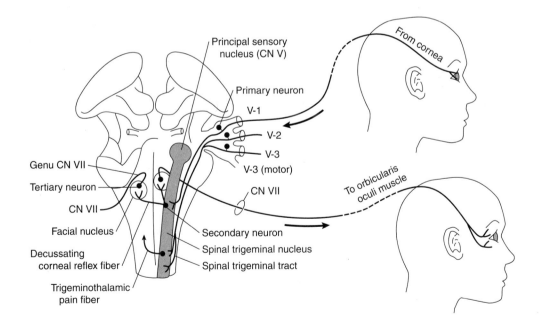

Figure 13-4.   The corneal reflex pathway showing the three neurons and decussation. This reflex is consensual, like the pupillary light reflex. Second-order pain neurons are found in the caudal division of the spinal trigeminal nucleus. Second-order corneal reflex neurons are found at more rostral levels.

VI. THE ABDUCENT NERVE (CN VI)

A. General characteristics. The abducent nerve is a pure **GSE nerve** that innervates the lateral rectus muscle, which abducts the eye.

    1. It arises from the abducent nucleus that is found in the dorsomedial tegmentum of the caudal pons.

    2. Exiting intraaxial fibers pass through the corticospinal tract. A **lesion** results in **alternating abducent hemiparesis.**

    3. It passes through the pontine cistern and cavernous sinus and enters the orbit through the superior orbital fissure.

B. Clinical correlation. CN VI paralysis is the most common isolated palsy that results from the long peripheral course of the nerve. It is seen in patients with meningitis, subarachnoid hemorrhage, late-stage syphilis, and trauma. **Abducent nerve paralysis** results in the **following defects:**

    1. Convergent (medial) strabismus (esotropia) with inability to abduct the eye

    2. Horizontal diplopia with maximum separation of the double images when looking toward the paretic lateral rectus muscle

VII. THE FACIAL NERVE (CN VII)

A. General characteristics. The facial nerve is a **GSA,** general visceral afferent **(GVA), SVA, GVE,** and **SVE** nerve (Figures 13-5 and 13-6). It **mediates facial movements, taste, salivation, lacrimation,** and **general sensation from the external ear.** It is the nerve of the pharyngeal (brachial) arch 2 (hyoid). It includes the facial nerve proper (motor division), which contains the SVE fibers that **innervate the muscles of facial**

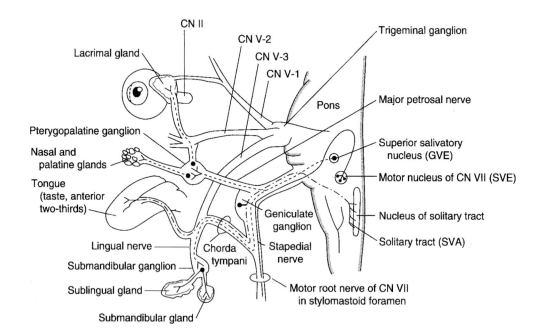

Figure 13-5. The functional components of the facial nerve [cranial nerve (CN) VII].

Face area of motor cortex

UMN lesion of corticobulbar tract (e.g., stroke of internal capsule)

Facial nucleus of pons

Upper face division

Lower face division

Muscles of facial expression:

Frontalis

Orbicularis oculi

Buccinator

Orbicularis oris

Platysma

LMN lesion of CN VII (e.g., Bell's palsy)

Figure 13-6.   Corticobulbar innervation of the facial nerve [cranial nerve (*CN*) VII] nucleus. An upper motor neuron (*UMN*) lesion (e.g., stroke involving the internal capsule) results in contralateral weakness of the lower face, with sparing of the upper face. A lower motor neuron (*LMN*) lesion (e.g., Bell's palsy) results in paralysis of the facial muscles in both the upper and lower face.

(mimetic) expression. CN VII includes the intermediate nerve, which contains GSA, SVA, and GVE fibers. All first-order sensory neurons are found in the geniculate ganglion within the temporal bone.

1. **Anatomy.** The facial nerve exits the brain stem in the cerebellopontine angle. It enters the internal auditory meatus and the facial canal. It then exits the facial canal and skull through the stylomastoid foramen.

2. The **GSA component** has cell bodies located in the geniculate ganglion. It innervates the posterior surface of the external ear through the posterior auricular branch of CN VII. It projects centrally to the spinal trigeminal tract and nucleus.

3. The **GVA component** has no clinical significance. The cell bodies are located in the geniculate ganglion. Fibers innervate the soft palate and the adjacent pharyngeal wall.

4. The **SVA component (taste)** has cell bodies located in the geniculate ganglion. It projects centrally to the solitary tract and nucleus. It innervates the taste buds from the anterior two-thirds of the tongue through:

   a. The **intermediate nerve**

   b. The **chorda tympani,** which is located in the tympanic cavity medial to the tympanic membrane and malleus. It contains the SVA and GVE (parasympathetic) fibers.

   c. The **lingual nerve** (a branch of CN V-3)

   d. The **central gustatory pathway** (see Figure 13-5). Taste fibers from CN VII, CN IX, and CN X project through the solitary tract to the solitary nucleus. The solitary nucleus projects through the central tegmental tract to the ventral posteromedial nucleus (VPM) of the thalamus. The VPM projects to the gustatory cortex of the parietal lobe (parietal operculum).

5. The **GVE component** is a parasympathetic component that innervates the lacrimal, submandibular, and sublingual glands. It contains preganglionic parasympathetic neurons that are located in the superior salivatory nucleus of the caudal pons.

   a. **Lacrimal pathway** (see Figure 13-5). The superior salivatory nucleus projects through the intermediate and greater petrosal nerves to the pterygopalatine (sphenopalatine) ganglion. The pterygopalatine ganglion projects to the lacrimal gland of the orbit.

   b. **Submandibular pathway** (see Figure 13-5). The superior salivatory nucleus projects through the intermediate nerve and chorda tympani to the submandibular ganglion. The submandibular ganglion projects to and innervates the submandibular and sublingual glands.

6. The **SVE component** arises from the facial nucleus, loops around the abducent nucleus of the caudal pons, and exits the brain stem in the cerebellopontine angle. It enters the internal auditory meatus, traverses the facial canal, sends a branch to the stapedius muscle of the middle ear, and exits the skull through the stylomastoid foramen. It innervates the muscles of facial expression, the stylohyoid muscle, the posterior belly of the digastric muscle, and the stapedius muscle.

B. **Clinical correlation. Lesions** (see Figure 14-2) cause the following conditions:

   1. **Flaccid paralysis** of the **muscles of facial expression** (upper and lower face)

   2. **Loss of the corneal reflex** (efferent limb), which may lead to corneal ulceration

   3. **Loss of taste** (ageusia-gustatory anesthesia) from the anterior two-thirds of the tongue, which may result from damage to the chorda tympani

   4. **Hyperacusis** (increased acuity to sounds) as a result of stapedius paralysis

   5. **Bell's palsy** (peripheral facial paralysis), which is caused by trauma or infection and involves the upper and lower face

   6. **Crocodile tears syndrome** (lacrimation during eating), which is a result of aberrant regeneration after trauma

   7. **Supranuclear (central) facial palsy,** which results in contralateral weakness of the lower face, with sparing of the upper face (see Figure 13-6)

   8. **Bilateral facial nerve palsies,** which occur in Guillain-Barré syndrome (see Chapter 14)

> **9. Möbius' syndrome,** which consists of congenital facial diplegia (CN VII) and convergent strabismus (CN VI)

VIII. **THE VESTIBULOCOCHLEAR NERVE (CN VIII)** is an SSA nerve. It has two functional divisions: the vestibular nerve, which **maintains equilibrium and balance,** and the cochlear nerve, which **mediates hearing** (see Chapters 11 and 12). It exits the brain stem at the cerebellopontine angle and enters the internal auditory meatus. It is confined to the temporal bone.

A. Vestibular nerve (see Figure 12-1)

1. General characteristics

   a. It is associated functionally with the cerebellum (flocculonodular lobe) and ocular motor nuclei.

   b. It regulates compensatory eye movements.

   c. Its first-order sensory bipolar neurons are located in the vestibular ganglion in the fundus of the internal auditory meatus.

   d. It projects its peripheral processes to the hair cells of the cristae of the semicircular ducts and the hair cells of the utricle and saccule.

   e. It projects its central processes to the four vestibular nuclei of the brain stem and the flocculonodular lobe of the cerebellum.

   f. It conducts efferent fibers to the hair cells from the brain stem.

2. **Clinical correlation. Lesions** result in **disequilibrium, vertigo,** and **nystagmus.**

B. Cochlear nerve (see Figure 11-1)

1. General characteristics

   a. Its first-order sensory bipolar neurons are located in the spiral (cochlear) ganglion of the modiolus of the cochlea, within the temporal bone.

   b. It projects its peripheral processes to the hair cells of the organ of Corti.

   c. It projects its central processes to the dorsal and ventral cochlear nuclei of the brain stem.

   d. It conducts efferent fibers to the hair cells from the brain stem.

2. **Clinical correlation.** Destructive lesions cause **hearing loss** (sensorineural deafness). Irritative lesions can cause **tinnitus** (ear ringing). An **acoustic neuroma** (schwannoma) is a Schwann cell tumor of the cochlear nerve that causes deafness (see Chapter 14).

IX. **THE GLOSSOPHARYNGEAL NERVE (CN IX)** is a GSA, GVA, SVA, SVE, and GVE nerve (Figure 13-7).

A. General characteristics. The glossopharyngeal nerve is primarily a sensory nerve. Along with CN X, CN XI, and CN XII, it **mediates taste, salivation,** and **swallowing.** It **mediates input** from the **carotid sinus,** which contains baroreceptors that monitor arterial blood pressure. It also **mediates input** from the **carotid body,** which contains chemoreceptors that monitor the CO_2 and O_2 concentration of the blood.

1. **Anatomy.** CN IX is the nerve of pharyngeal (branchial) arch 3. It exits the brain stem (medulla) from the postolivary sulcus with CN X and CN XI. It exits the skull through the jugular foramen with CN X and CN XI.

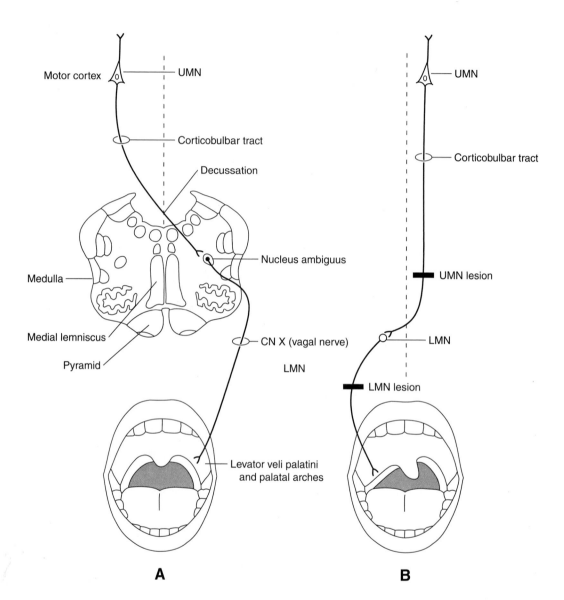

Motor cortex — UMN

Corticobulbar tract

Decussation

Nucleus ambiguus

Medulla

Medial lemniscus

Pyramid

CN X (vagal nerve)

LMN

Levator veli palatini
and palatal arches

UMN

Corticobulbar tract

UMN lesion

LMN

LMN lesion

A   **B**

Figure 13-7.   Innervation of the palatal arches and uvula. Sensory innervation is mediated by the glossopharyngeal nerve [cranial nerve (CN) IX]. Motor innervation of the palatal arches and uvula is mediated by the vagus nerve (CN X). (A) A normal palate and uvula in a person who is saying "Ah." (B) A patient with an upper motor neuron (UMN) lesion (left) and a lower motor neuron (LMN) lesion (right). When this patient says "Ah," the palatal arches sag. The uvula deviates toward the intact (left) side.

   2. The **GSA component** innervates part of the external ear and the external auditory meatus through the auricular branch of the vagus nerve. It has cell bodies in the superior ganglion. It projects its central processes to the spinal trigeminal tract and nucleus.

   3. The **GVA component** innervates structures that are derived from the endoderm (e.g., pharynx). It **innervates** the **mucous membranes** of the posterior one-third of the tongue, tonsil, upper pharynx, tympanic cavity, and auditory tube. It also **innervates** the **carotid sinus** (baroreceptors) and **carotid body** (chemoreceptors) through the sinus nerve. It has cell bodies in the inferior (petrosal) ganglion. It is the afferent limb of the gag reflex and the carotid sinus reflex.

   4. The **SVA component** innervates the taste buds of the posterior one-third of the tongue. It has cell bodies in the inferior (petrosal) ganglion. It projects its central processes to the solitary tract and nucleus (for a discussion of the central pathway, see VII A 4 d).

   5. The **SVE component** innervates only the stylopharyngeus muscle. It arises from the nucleus ambiguus of the lateral medulla.

   6. The **GVE component** is a parasympathetic component that innervates the parotid gland. Preganglionic parasympathetic neurons are located in the inferior salivatory nucleus of the medulla. They project through the tympanic and lesser petrosal nerves to the otic ganglion. Postganglionic fibers from the otic ganglion project to the parotid gland through the auriculotemporal nerve (CN V-3).

B. **Clinical correlation. Lesions** cause the following conditions:

   1. **Loss of the gag (pharyngeal) reflex** (interruption of the afferent limb)

   2. **Hypersensitive carotid sinus reflex** (syncope)

   3. **Loss of general sensation** in the **pharynx, tonsils, fauces,** and **back of the tongue**

   4. **Loss of taste** from the posterior one-third of the tongue

   5. **Glossopharyngeal neuralgia,** which is characterized by severe stabbing pain in the root of the tongue

X. THE VAGAL NERVE (CN X) is a GSA, GVA, SVA, SVE, and GVE nerve (see Figure 13-7).

A. **General characteristics.** The vagal nerve **mediates phonation, swallowing** (with CN IX, CN XI, and CN XII), elevation of the palate, taste, and cutaneous sensation from the ear. **It innervates the viscera** of the **neck, thorax,** and **abdomen.**

   1. **Anatomy.** The vagal nerve is the nerve of pharyngeal (brachial) arches 4 and 6. Pharyngeal arch 5 is either absent or rudimentary. It exits the brain stem (medulla) from the postolivary sulcus. It exits the skull through the jugular foramen with CN IX and CN XI.

   2. The **GSA component** innervates the infratentorial dura, external ear, external auditory meatus, and tympanic membrane. It has cell bodies in the superior (jugular) ganglion, and it projects its central processes to the spinal trigeminal tract and nucleus.

   3. The **GVA component** innervates the mucous membranes of the pharynx, larynx, esophagus, trachea, and thoracic and abdominal viscera (to the left colic flexure).

It has cell bodies in the inferior (nodose) ganglion. It projects its central processes to the solitary tract and nucleus.

4. The **SVA component** innervates the taste buds in the epiglottic region. It has cell bodies in the inferior (nodose) ganglion. It projects its central processes to the solitary tract and nucleus. For a discussion of the central pathway, see VII A 4 d.

5. The **SVE component** innervates the pharyngeal (brachial) arch muscles of the larynx and pharynx, the striated muscle of the upper esophagus, the muscle of the uvula, and the levator veli palatini and palatoglossus muscles. It receives SVE input from the cranial division of the spinal accessory nerve (CN XI). It arises from the nucleus ambiguus in the lateral medulla. The SVE component provides the efferent limb of the gag reflex.

6. The **GVE component** innervates the viscera of the neck and the thoracic (heart) and abdominal cavities as far as the left colic flexure. Preganglionic parasympathetic neurons that are located in the dorsal motor nucleus of the medulla project to the terminal (intramural) ganglia of the visceral organs (see Figure 18-2 and Table 18-1).

B. Clinical correlation. Lesions and **reflexes** cause the following conditions:

1. Ipsilateral paralysis of the soft palate, pharynx, and larynx that leads to dysphonia (hoarseness), dyspnea, dysarthria, and dysphagia

2. Loss of the gag (palatal) reflex (efferent limb)

3. Anesthesia of the pharynx and larynx that leads to unilateral loss of the cough reflex

4. Aortic aneurysms and tumors of the neck and thorax that frequently compress the vagal nerve

5. Complete laryngeal paralysis, which can be rapidly fatal if it is bilateral (asphyxia)

6. Parasympathetic (vegetative) disturbances, including bradycardia (irritative lesion), tachycardia (destructive lesion), and dilation of the stomach

7. The **oculocardiac reflex,** in which pressure on the eye slows the heart rate (afferent limb of CN V-1 and efferent limb of CN X)

8. The **carotid sinus reflex,** in which pressure on the carotid sinus slows the heart rate (bradycardia) [efferent limb of CN X]

XI. THE ACCESSORY NERVE (CN XI), or **spinal accessory nerve,** is an SVE nerve (Figure 13-8).

A. General characteristics. The accessory nerve **mediates head and shoulder movement** and **innervates** the **laryngeal muscles.** It has the following divisions:

1. The **cranial division (accessory portion),** which arises from the nucleus ambiguus of the medulla. It exits the medulla from the postolivary sulcus and joins the vagal nerve (CN X). It exits the skull through the jugular foramen with CN IX and CN X. It **innervates** the **intrinsic muscles** of the **larynx** through the inferior (recurrent) laryngeal nerve, with the exception of the cricothyroid muscle.

2. The **spinal division (spinal portion),** which arises from the ventral horn of cervical segments C1 through C6. The spinal roots exit the spinal cord laterally between the ventral and dorsal spinal roots, ascend through the foramen magnum, and

Figure 13-8.   The cranial and spinal divisions of the accessory nerve [cranial nerve (CN) XI]. The cranial division hitchhikes a ride with the accessory nerve, then joins the vagal nerve to become the inferior (recurrent) laryngeal nerve. The recurrent laryngeal nerve innervates the intrinsic muscles of the larynx, except for the cricothyroid muscle. The spinal division innervates the trapezoid and sternocleidomastoid muscles. Three nerves pass through the jugular foramen (glomus jugulare tumor).

exit the skull through the jugular foramen. It **innervates** the **sternocleidomastoid muscle** with the cervical plexus (C-2) and the **trapezius muscle** with the cervical plexus (C-3 and C-4).

B. Clinical correlation. Lesions cause the following conditions:

1. Paralysis of the sternocleidomastoid muscle that results in difficulty in turning the head to the contralateral side

2. Paralysis of the trapezius muscle that results in shoulder droop and inability to shrug the shoulder

3. Paralysis of the larynx if the cranial root is involved

XII. THE HYPOGLOSSAL NERVE (CN XII) is a GSE nerve (Figure 13-9).

A. General characteristics. The hypoglossal nerve **mediates tongue movement.** It arises from the hypoglossal nucleus of the medulla and exits the medulla in the preolivary sulcus. It exits the skull through the hypoglossal canal, and it **innervates** the **intrinsic and extrinsic muscles** of the **tongue.** Extrinsic muscles are the genioglossus, styloglossus, and hyoglossus.

B. Clinical correlation

1. Transection results in hemiparalysis of the tongue.

2. Protrusion causes the tongue to point toward the weak side because of the unopposed action of the opposite genioglossus muscle (Figure 13-10).

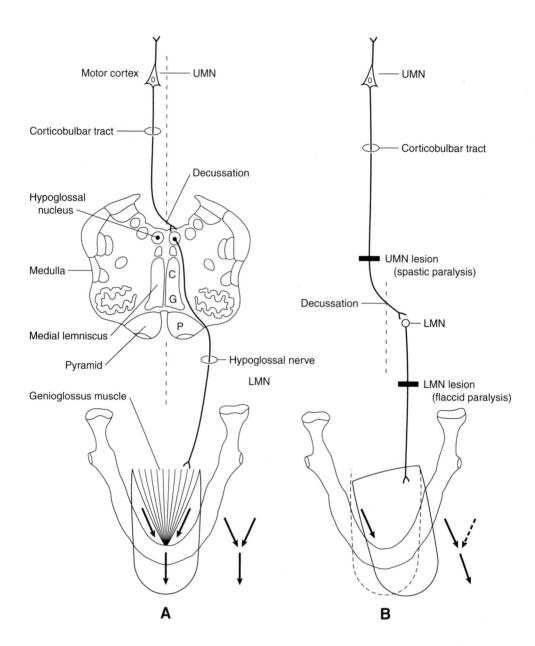

Figure 13-9. Motor innervation of the tongue. Corticobulbar fibers project predominantly to the contralateral hypoglossal nucleus. An upper motor neuron (*UMN*) lesion causes deviation of the protruded tongue to the weak (contralateral) side. A lower motor neuron (*LMN*) lesion causes deviation of the protruded tongue to the weak (ipsilateral) side. (A) Normal tongue. (B) Tongue with UMN and LMN lesions.

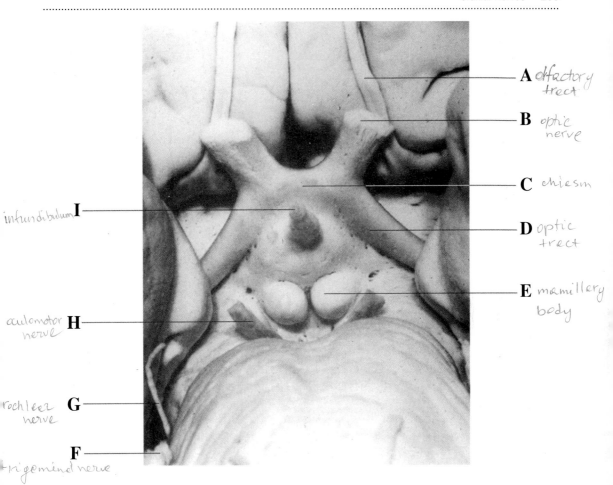

A olfactory trect

B optic nerve

C chiesm

D optic trect

E mamillary body

infundibulum **I**

oculomotor **H** nerve

trochleer **G** nerve

F

trigemind nerve

Figure 13-10. The basis cerebri showing cranial nerves and the floor of the hypothalamus: olfactory tract (A); optic nerve (B); chiasm (C); optic tract (D); mamillary body (E); trigeminal nerve (F); trochlear nerve (G); oculomotor nerve (H); infundibulum (I). (Reprinted with permission from Fix JD: *BRS Neuroanatomy*, 3rd ed. Baltimore, Williams & Wilkins, 1996, p. 293.)

14

Lesions of the Brain Stem

I. **LESIONS OF THE MEDULLA** (Figure 14-1)

A. **Medial medullary syndrome (anterior spinal artery syndrome).** Affected structures and resultant deficits include:

1. The **corticospinal tract** (medullary pyramid). Lesions result in contralateral spastic hemiparesis.

2. The **medial lemniscus.** Lesions result in contralateral loss of tactile and vibration sensation from the trunk and extremities.

3. The **hypoglossal nucleus or intraaxial root fibers [cranial nerve (CN) XII].** Lesions result in ipsilateral flaccid hemiparalysis of the tongue. When protruded, the tongue points to the side of the lesion (i.e., the weak side). See Figure 13-7.

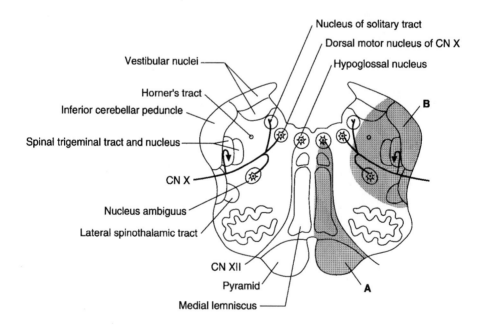

Figure 14-1. Vascular lesions of the caudal pons at the level of the hypoglossal nucleus of cranial nerve (CN) XII and the dorsal motor nucleus of CN X. (A) Medial medullary syndrome (arterial spinal artery). (B) Lateral medullary [posterior inferior cerebellar artery (PICA)] syndrome.

B. Lateral medullary syndrome [posterior inferior cerebellar artery (PICA) syn-drome] is characterized by dissociated sensory loss (see I B 6–7). Affected structures and resultant deficits include:

1. The **vestibular nuclei.** Lesions result in nystagmus, nausea, vomiting, and vertigo.

2. The **inferior cerebellar peduncle.** Lesions result in ipsilateral cerebellar signs [e.g., dystaxia, dysmetria (past pointing), dysdiadochokinesia].

3. The **nucleus ambiguus of CN IX, CN X, and CN XI.** Lesions result in ipsilateral laryngeal, pharyngeal, and palatal hemiparalysis [i.e., loss of the gag reflex (efferent limb), dysarthria, dysphagia, and dysphonia (hoarseness)].

4. The **glossopharyngeal nerve roots.** Lesions result in loss of the gag reflex (afferent limb).

5. The **vagal nerve roots.** Lesions result in the same deficits as seen in lesions involving the nucleus ambiguus (see I B 3).

6. The **spinothalamic tracts (spinal lemniscus).** Lesions result in contralateral loss of pain and temperature sensation from the trunk and extremities.

7. The **spinal trigeminal nucleus and tract.** Lesions result in ipsilateral loss of pain and temperature sensation from the face (facial hemianesthesia).

8. The **descending sympathetic tract.** Lesions result in ipsilateral Horner's syndrome (i.e., ptosis, miosis, hemianhidrosis, and apparent enophthalmos).

II. LESIONS OF THE PONS (Figure 14-2A)

A. Medial inferior pontine syndrome results from occlusion of the paramedian branches of the basilar artery. Affected structures and resultant deficits include:

1. The **corticospinal tract.** Lesions result in contralateral spastic hemiparesis.

2. The **medial lemniscus.** Lesions result in contralateral loss of tactile sensation from the trunk and extremities.

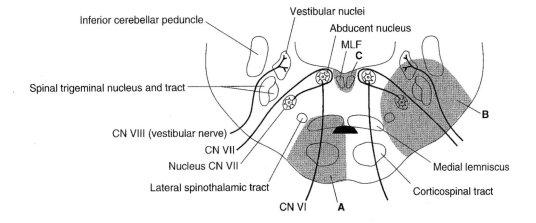

Figure 14-2. Vascular lesions of the caudal pons at the level of the abducent nucleus of cranial nerve (CN) VI and the facial nucleus of CN VII. (A) Medial inferior pontine syndrome. (B) Lateral inferior pontine syndrome [anterior inferior cerebellar artery (AICA) syndrome]. (C) Medial longitudinal fasciculus (MLF) syndrome.

3. The **abducent nerve roots.** Lesions result in ipsilateral lateral rectus paralysis.

B. **Lateral inferior pontine syndrome** [anterior inferior cerebellar artery (AICA) syndrome] (Figure 14-2B). Affected structures and resultant deficits include:

1. The **facial nucleus and intraaxial nerve fibers.** Lesions result in:

a. Ipsilateral facial nerve paralysis

b. Ipsilateral loss of taste from the anterior two-thirds of the tongue

c. Ipsilateral loss of lacrimation and reduced salivation

d. Loss of corneal and stapedial reflexes (efferent limbs)

2. The **cochlear nuclei and intraaxial nerve fibers.** Lesions result in unilateral central deafness.

3. The **vestibular nuclei and intraaxial nerve fibers.** Lesions result in nystagmus, nausea, vomiting, and vertigo.

4. The **spinal trigeminal nucleus and tract.** Lesions result in ipsilateral loss of pain and temperature sensation from the face (facial hemianesthesia).

5. The **middle and inferior cerebellar peduncles.** Lesions result in ipsilateral limb and gait dystaxia.

6. The **spinothalamic tracts (spinal lemniscus).** Lesions result in contralateral loss of pain and temperature sensation from the trunk and extremities.

7. The **descending sympathetic tract.** Lesions result in ipsilateral Horner's syndrome.

C. **Medial longitudinal fasciculus (MLF) syndrome (internuclear ophthalmoplegia)** [see Figure 14-2C] interrupts fibers from the contralateral abducent nucleus that project through the MLF to the ipsilateral medial rectus subnucleus of CN III. It causes **medial rectus palsy** on attempted lateral conjugate gaze and **nystagmus** in the abducting eye. Convergence remains intact. This syndrome is often seen in patients with **multiple sclerosis.**

D. **Facial colliculus syndrome** usually results from a pontine glioma or a vascular accident. The internal genu of CN VII and the nucleus of CN VI underlie the facial colliculus.

1. Lesions of the **internal genu** of the **facial nerve** cause:

a. Ipsilateral facial paralysis

b. Ipsilateral loss of the corneal reflex

2. Lesions of the **abducent nucleus** cause:

a. Lateral rectus paralysis

b. Medial (convergent) strabismus

c. Horizontal diplopia

III. LESIONS OF THE MIDBRAIN (Figure 14-3)

A. **Dorsal midbrain (Parinaud's) syndrome** (see Figure 14-3A) is often the result of a pinealoma or germinoma of the pineal region. Affected structures and resultant deficits include:

1. The **superior colliculus** and **pretectal area.** Lesions cause paralysis of upward and downward gaze, pupillary disturbances, and absence of convergence.

2. The **cerebral aqueduct.** Compression causes noncommunicating hydrocephalus.

B. **Paramedian midbrain (Benedikt) syndrome** (see Figure 14-3B). Affected structures and resultant deficits include:

Figure 14-3.   Lesions of the rostral midbrain at the level of the superior colliculus and oculomotor nucleus of cranial nerve (CN) III. (A) Dorsal midbrain (Parinaud's) syndrome. (B) Paramedian midbrain (Benedikt) syndrome. (C) Medial midbrain (Weber) syndrome.

1. The **oculomotor nerve roots** (intraaxial fibers). Lesions cause complete ipsilateral oculomotor paralysis. Eye abduction and depression is caused by the intact lateral rectus (CN VI) and superior oblique (CN IV) muscles. Ptosis (paralysis of the levator palpebra muscle) and fixation and dilation of the ipsilateral pupil (complete internal ophthalmoplegia) also occur.

2. The **dentatothalamic fibers.** Lesions cause contralateral cerebellar dystaxia with intention tremor.

3. The **medial lemniscus.** Lesions result in contralateral loss of tactile sensation from the trunk and extremities.

C. **Medial midbrain (Weber) syndrome** (see Figure 14-3C). Affected structures and resultant deficits include:

1. The **oculomotor nerve roots** (intraaxial fibers). Lesions cause complete ipsilateral oculomotor paralysis. Eye abduction and depression are caused by intact lateral rectus (CN VI) and superior oblique (CN IV) muscles. Ptosis and fixation and dilation of the ipsilateral pupil also occur.

2. The **corticospinal tracts.** Lesions result in contralateral spastic hemiparesis.

3. The **corticobulbar fibers.** Lesions cause contralateral weakness of the lower face (CN VII), tongue (CN XII), and palate (CN X). The upper face division of the facial nucleus receives bilateral corticobulbar input. The uvula and pharyngeal wall are pulled toward the normal side (CN X), and the protruded tongue points to the weak side.

IV. **ACOUSTIC NEUROMA (SCHWANNOMA)** [Figure 14-4] is a benign tumor of Schwann cells that affects the vestibulocochlear nerve (CN VIII). It accounts for 8% of all intracranial tumors. It is a posterior fossa tumor of the internal auditory meatus and cerebellopontine angle. The neuroma often compresses the facial nerve (CN VII), which accompanies CN VIII in the cerebellopontine angle and internal auditory meatus. It may impinge on the pons and affect the spinal trigeminal tract (CN V). **Schwannomas** occur twice as often in females as in males. Affected structures and resultant deficits include:

Figure 14-4. Magnetic resonance image of an acoustic neuroma. This coronal section shows dilation of the ventricles. The vestibulocochlear nerve is visible in the left internal auditory meatus. The tumor indents the lateral pons. Cranial nerve (CN) palsies include CN V, VII, and VIII. Symptoms include unilateral deafness, facial anesthesia and weakness, and an absent coronal reflex. This is a T1-weighted image.

A. The **cochlear nerve of CN VIII.** Damage results in tinnitus and unilateral nerve deafness.

B. The **vestibular nerve of CN VIII.** Damage results in vertigo, nystagmus, nausea, vomiting, and unsteadiness of gait.

C. The **facial nerve (CN VII).** Damage results in facial weakness and loss of the corneal reflex (efferent limb).

D. The **spinal trigeminal tract (CN V).** Damage results in paresthesia, anesthesia of the ipsilateral face, and loss of the corneal reflex (afferent limb).

E. **Neurofibromatosis type 2** often occurs with bilateral acoustic neuromas.

V. **JUGULAR FORAMEN SYNDROME** usually results from a posterior fossa tumor (e.g., **glomus jugulare tumor,** the most common inner ear tumor) that compresses CN IX, X, and XI. Affected structures and resultant deficits include:

A. The **glossopharyngeal nerve** (CN IX). Damage results in:

   1. Ipsilateral loss of the gag reflex

   2. Ipsilateral loss of pain, temperature, and taste in the tongue

B. The **vagal nerve** (CN X). Damage results in:

   1. Ipsilateral paralysis of the soft palate and larynx

   2. Ipsilateral loss of the gag reflex

C. The **accessory nerve** (CN XI). Damage results in:

1. Paralysis of the sternocleidomastoid muscle, which results in the inability to turn the head to the opposite side

2. Paralysis of the trapezius muscle, which causes shoulder droop and inability to shrug the shoulder

VI. "LOCKED-IN" SYNDROME is a lesion of the base of the pons as the result of infarction, trauma, tumor, or demyelination. The corticospinal and corticobulbar tracts are affected

Figure 14-5. Anatomy of the subclavian steal syndrome. Thrombosis of the proximal part of the subclavian artery (*left*) results in retrograde blood flow through the ipsilateral vertebral artery and into the left subclavian artery. Blood can be shunted from the right vertebral artery and down the left vertebral artery (A). Blood may also reach the left vertebral artery through the carotid circulation (B). ACA = anterior cerebellar artery; ACOM = anterior communicating artery; AICA = anterior inferior cerebellar artery; ASA = anterior spinal artery; BA = basilar artery; BCT = brachiocephalic trunk; CCA = common carotid artery; ECA = external carotid artery; ICA = internal carotid artery; MCA = middle cerebral artery; PCA = posterior cerebral artery; PCOM = posterior communicating artery; PICA = posterior inferior cerebellar artery; SCA = superior communicating artery; SCLA = subclavian artery; VA = vertebral artery.

bilaterally. The oculomotor and trochlear nerves are not injured. Patients are conscious and may communicate through vertical eye movements.

VII. **CENTRAL PONTINE MYELINOLYSIS** is a lesion of the base of the pons that affects the corticospinal and corticobulbar tracts. More than 75% of cases are associated with alcoholism or rapid correction of hyponatremia. Symptoms include spastic quadriparesis, pseudobulbar palsy, and mental changes. This condition may become the locked-in syndrome.

VIII. **"TOP OF THE BASILAR" SYNDROME** results from embolic occlusion of the rostral basilar artery. Neurologic signs include optic ataxia and psychic paralysis of fixation of gaze **(Balint's syndrome),** ectopic pupils, somnolence, and cortical blindness, with or without visual anosognosia **(Anton's syndrome).**

IX. **SUBCLAVIAN STEAL SYNDROME** (Figure 14-5) results from thrombosis of the left subclavian artery proximal to the vertebral artery. Blood is shunted retrograde down the left vertebral artery and into the left subclavian artery. Clinical signs include transient weakness and claudication of the left arm on exercise and vertebrobasilar insufficiency (i.e., vertigo, dizziness).

X. **THE CEREBELLOPONTINE ANGLE** is the junction of the medulla, pons, and cerebellum. CN VII and VIII are found there. Five brain tumors, including a cyst, are often located in the cerebellopontine angle cistern. Remember the acronym **SAME:** **s**chwannoma **(75%), a**rachnoid cyst **(1%), m**eningioma **(10%), e**pendymoma **(1%),** and epidermoid **(5%).** The percentages refer to cerebellopontine angle tumors.

15

Cerebellum

I. FUNCTION. The cerebellum has three primary functions:

A. Maintenance of posture and balance

B. Maintenance of muscle tone

C. Coordination of voluntary motor activity

II. ANATOMY

A. Cerebellar peduncles

    1. The **superior cerebellar peduncle** contains the major output from the cerebellum, the dentatothalamic tract. This tract terminates in the ventral lateral nucleus of the thalamus. It has one major afferent pathway, the ventral spinocerebellar tract.

    2. The **middle cerebellar peduncle** receives pontocerebellar fibers, which project to the neocerebellum (pontocerebellum).

    3. The **inferior cerebellar peduncle** has three major afferent tracts: the dorsal spinocerebellar tract, the cuneocerebellar tract, and the olivocerebellar tract from the contralateral inferior olivary nucleus.

B. Cerebellar cortex, neurons, and fibers

    1. The cerebellar cortex has three layers.

        a. The **molecular layer** is the outer layer underlying the pia. It contains stellate cells, basket cells, and the dendritic arbor of the Purkinje cells.

        b. The **Purkinje cell layer** lies between the molecular and the granule cell layers.

        c. The **granule layer** is the inner layer overlying the white matter. It contains granule cells, Golgi cells, and cerebellar glomeruli. A cerebellar glomerulus consists of a mossy fiber rosette, granule cell dendrites, and a Golgi cell axon.

    2. Neurons and fibers of the cerebellum

        a. Purkinje cells convey the only output from the cerebellar cortex. They project inhibitory output [i.e., γ-aminobutyric acid (GABA)] to the cerebellar and vestibular nuclei. These cells are excited by parallel and climbing fibers and inhibited by GABA-ergic basket and stellate cells.

        b. Granule cells excite (by way of glutamate) Purkinje, basket, stellate, and Golgi cells through parallel fibers. They are inhibited by Golgi cells and excited by mossy fibers.

c. **Parallel fibers** are the axons of granule cells. These fibers extend into the molecular layer.

d. **Mossy fibers** are the afferent excitatory fibers of the spinocerebellar, ponto-cerebellar, and vestibulocerebellar tracts. They terminate as mossy fiber ro-settes on granule cell dendrites. They excite granule cells to discharge through their parallel fibers.

e. **Climbing fibers** are the afferent excitatory (by way of aspartate) fibers of the olivocerebellar tract. These fibers arise from the contralateral inferior olivary nucleus. They terminate on neurons of the cerebellar nuclei and dendrites of Purkinje cells.

III. THE MAJOR CEREBELLAR PATHWAY (Figure 15-1) consists of the following structures.

A. The **Purkinje cells of the cerebellar cortex** project to the cerebellar nuclei (e.g., dentate, emboliform, globose, and fastigial nuclei).

Figure 15-1.   The principal cerebellar connections. The major efferent pathway is the dentatothalamocorti-cal tract. The cerebellum receives input from the cerebral cortex through the corticopontocerebellar tract.

B. The **dentate nucleus** is the major effector nucleus of the cerebellum. It gives rise to the dentatothalamic tract, which projects through the superior cerebellar peduncle to the contralateral ventral lateral nucleus of the thalamus. The decussation of the superior cerebellar peduncle is in the caudal midbrain tegmentum.

C. The **ventral lateral nucleus of the thalamus** receives the dentatothalamic tract. It projects to the primary motor cortex of the precentral gyrus (Brodmann's area 4).

D. The **motor cortex (motor strip, or Brodmann's area 4)** receives input from the ventral lateral nucleus of the thalamus. It projects as the corticopontine tract to the pontine nuclei.

E. The **pontine nuclei** receive input from the motor cortex. Axons project as the pontocerebellar tract to the contralateral cerebellar cortex, where they terminate as mossy fibers, thus completing the circuit.

IV. CEREBELLAR DYSFUNCTION includes the following triad:

A. **Hypotonia** is loss of the resistance normally offered by muscles to palpation or passive manipulation. It results in a floppy, loose-jointed, rag-doll appearance with pendular reflexes. The patient appears inebriated.

B. **Dysequilibrium** is loss of balance characterized by gait and trunk dystaxia.

C. **Dyssynergia** is loss of coordinated muscle activity. It includes **dysmetria, intention tremor, failure to check movements, nystagmus, dysdiadochokinesia,** and **dysrhythmokinesia. Cerebellar nystagmus** is **coarse.** It is **more pronounced when the patient looks toward the side of the lesion.**

V. CEREBELLAR SYNDROMES AND TUMORS (Figure 15-2)

A. **Anterior vermis syndrome** involves the leg region of the anterior lobe. It results from atrophy of the rostral vermis, most commonly caused by alcohol abuse. It causes gait, trunk, and leg dystaxia.

B. **Posterior vermis syndrome** involves the flocculonodular lobe. It is usually the result of brain tumors in children and is most commonly caused by medulloblastomas or ependymomas. It causes truncal dystaxia.

C. **Hemispheric syndrome** usually involves one cerebellar hemisphere. It is often the result of a brain tumor (astrocytoma) or an abscess (secondary to otitis media or mastoiditis). It causes arm, leg, and gait dystaxia and ipsilateral cerebellar signs.

D. **Cerebellar tumors.** In children, 70% of brain tumors are found in the posterior fossa. In adults, 70% of brain tumors are found in the supratentorial compartment.

1. **Astrocytomas** constitute 30% of all brain tumors in children. They are most often found in the cerebellar hemisphere. After surgical removal, it is common for the child to survive for many years.

2. **Medulloblastomas** are malignant and constitute 20% of all brain tumors in children. They are believed to originate from the superficial granule layer of the cerebellar cortex. They usually obstruct the passage of cerebrospinal fluid (CSF). As a result, hydrocephalus occurs.

3. **Ependymomas** constitute 15% of all brain tumors in children. They occur most frequently in the fourth ventricle. They usually obstruct the passage of CSF and cause hydrocephalus.

Figure 15-2.   Various forms of cerebellar atrophy. Abbreviations: MCP = middle cerebellar peduncle, ICP = inferior cerebellar peduncle, SCP = superior cerebellar peduncle. (Reprinted with permission from Poirier J, Gray F, Escourolle R: *Manual of Basic Neuropathology,* 3rd ed. Philadelphia, WB Saunders, 1990, p. 155.) (*Figure continues.*)

E Olivopontocerebellar atrophy

F Dentatorubral atrophy

Figure 15-2. Continued.

16
Thalamus

I. INTRODUCTION. The thalamus is the largest division of the diencephalon. It plays an important role in the integration of the sensory and motor systems.

II. MAJOR THALAMIC NUCLEI AND THEIR CONNECTIONS (Figure 16-1)

   A. The **anterior nucleus** receives hypothalamic input from the mamillary nucleus through the mamillothalamic tract. It projects to the cingulate gyrus and is part of the Papez circuit of emotion of the limbic system.

   B. The **mediodorsal (dorsomedial) nucleus** is reciprocally connected to the prefrontal cortex. It has abundant connections with intralaminar nuclei. It receives input from the amygdala, substantia nigra, and temporal neocortex. When it is destroyed, **memory loss** occurs (Wernicke-Korsakoff syndrome). The mediodorsal nucleus plays a role in the expression of affect, emotion, and behavior (limbic function).

   C. The **centromedian nucleus** is the largest intralaminar nucleus. It is reciprocally connected to the motor cortex (Brodmann's area 4). The centromedian nucleus receives input from the globus pallidus. It projects to the striatum (caudate nucleus and putamen) and projects diffusely to the entire neocortex.

   D. The **pulvinar** is the largest thalamic nucleus. It has reciprocal connections with the association cortex of the occipital, parietal, and posterior temporal lobes. It receives input from the lateral and medial geniculate bodies and the superior colliculus. It plays a role in the **integration of visual, auditory, and somesthetic input.** Destruction of the dominant pulvinar may result in sensory dysphasia.

   E. Ventral tier nuclei

      1. The **ventral anterior nucleus** receives input from the globus pallidus and substantia nigra. It projects diffusely to the prefrontal cortex, orbital cortex, and premotor cortex (Brodmann's area 6).

      2. The **ventral lateral nucleus** receives input from the cerebellum (dentate nucleus), globus pallidus, and substantia nigra. It projects to the motor cortex (Brodmann's area 4) and the supplementary motor cortex (Brodmann's area 6).

      3. The **ventral posterior nucleus** (ventrobasal complex) is the nucleus of termination of general somatic afferent (touch, pain, and temperature) and special visceral afferent (taste) fibers. It has two subnuclei.

         a. The **ventral posterolateral nucleus** receives the spinothalamic tracts and the medial lemniscus. It projects to the somesthetic (sensory) cortex (Brodmann's areas 3, 1, and 2).

         b. The **ventral posteromedial (VPM) nucleus** receives the trigeminothalamic tracts and projects to the somesthetic (sensory) cortex (Brodmann's areas 3, 1, and 2). The gustatory (taste) pathway originates in the solitary nucleus and

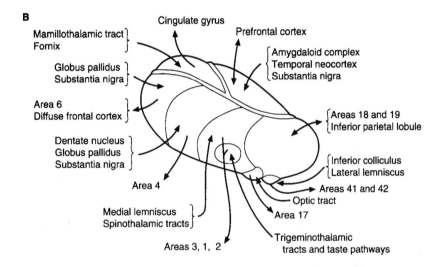

Figure 16-1. Major thalamic nuclei and their connections. (A) Dorsolateral aspect and major nuclei. (B) Major afferent and efferent connections. VA = ventral anterior nucleus; VL = ventral lateral nucleus; VPL = ventral posterior lateral nucleus; VPM = ventral posterior medial nucleus.

projects via the central tegmental tract to VPM, and thence to the gustatory cortex of the postcentral gyrus (Brodmann's area 3b), of the frontal operculum and insular cortex. The taste pathway is ipsilateral.

F. Metathalamus

    1. The **lateral geniculate body** is a visual relay nucleus. It receives retinal input through the optic tract and projects to the primary visual cortex (Brodmann's area 17).

    2. The **medial geniculate body** is an auditory relay nucleus. It receives auditory input through the brachium of the inferior colliculus and projects to the primary auditory cortex (Brodmann's areas 41 and 42).

G. The **reticular nucleus of thalamus** surrounds the thalamus as a thin layer of γ-amino-butyric acid (GABA)-ergic neurons. It lies between the external medullary lamina and the internal capsule. It receives excitatory collateral input from corticothalamic and thalamocortical fibers. It projects inhibitory fibers to thalamic nuclei from which it receives input. It is thought to play a role in normal electroencephaolgram readings.

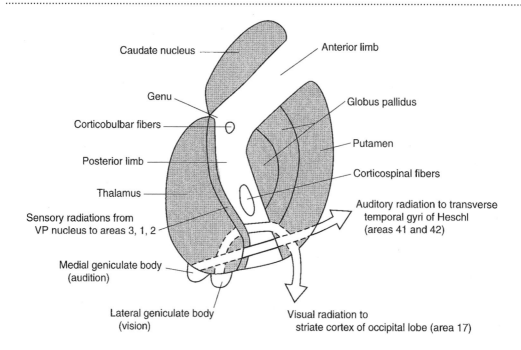

Figure 16-2. Horizontal section of the right internal capsule showing the major fiber projections. Clinically important tracts lie in the genu and posterior limb. Lesions of the internal capsule cause contralateral hemiparesis and contralateral hemianopia. *VP* = ventral posterior nucleus.

III. BLOOD SUPPLY. The thalamus is irrigated by three arteries (see Figure 3-3).

   A. The **posterior communicating artery**

   B. The **posterior cerebral artery**

   C. The **anterior choroidal artery** (lateral geniculate body)

IV. THE INTERNAL CAPSULE (Figure 16-2) is a layer of white matter (myelinated axons) that separates the caudate nucleus and the thalamus medially from the lentiform nucleus laterally.

   A. The **anterior limb** is located between the caudate nucleus and the lentiform nucleus (globus pallidus and putamen).

   B. The **genu** contains the corticobulbar fibers.

   C. The **posterior limb** is located between the thalamus and the lentiform nucleus. It contains corticospinal (pyramid) fibers as well as sensory (pain, temperature, and touch), visual, and auditory radiations.

   D. Blood supply

   1. The **anterior limb** is irrigated by the medial striate branches of the anterior cerebral artery and the lateral striate (lenticulostriate) branches of the middle cerebral artery.

   2. The **genu** is perfused either by direct branches from the internal carotid artery or by pallidal branches of the anterior choroidal artery.

   3. The **posterior limb** is supplied by branches of the anterior choroidal artery and lenticulostriate branches of the middle cerebral arteries.

17

Visual System

I. INTRODUCTION. The visual system is served by the optic nerve, which is a special somatic afferent nerve.

II. THE VISUAL PATHWAY (Figure 17-1) includes the following structures.

   A. Ganglion cells of the retina form the optic nerve [cranial nerve (CN) II]. They project from the nasal hemiretina to the contralateral lateral geniculate body and from the temporal hemiretina to the ipsilateral lateral geniculate body.

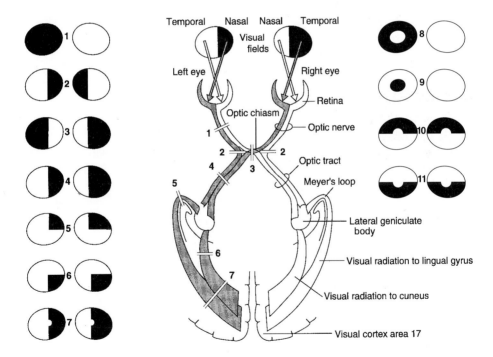

Figure 17-1. The visual pathway from the retina to the visual cortex showing visual field defects. (*1*) Ipsilateral blindness. (*2*) Binasal hemianopia. (*3*) Bitemporal hemianopia. (*4*) Right hemianopia. (*5*) Right upper quadrantanopia. (*6*) Right lower quadrantanopia. (*7*) Right hemianopia with macular sparing. (*8*) Left constricted field as a result of end-stage glaucoma. Bilateral constricted fields may be seen in hysteria. (*9*) Left central scotoma as seen in optic (retrobulbar) neuritis in multiple sclerosis. (*10*) Upper altitudinal hemianopia as a result of bilateral destruction of the lingual gyri. (*11*) Lower altitudinal hemianopia as a result of bilateral destruction of the cunei.

Figure 17-2. Histology of the retina. The retina has 10 layers: (*1*) pigment epithelium layer (PEL), (*2*) layer of rods and cones (LRC), (*3*) outer limiting membrane (OLM), (*4*) outer nuclear layer (ONL), (*5*) outer plexiform layer (OPL), (*6*) inner nuclear layer (INL), (*7*) inner plexiform layer (IPL), (*8*) ganglion cell layer (GCL), (*9*) nerve fiber layer (NFL), and (*10*) inner limiting layer (ILL). The tight junctions binding the pigment epithelial cells make up the blood-retina barrier. Retinal detachment usually occurs between the pigment layer and the layer of rods and cones. The central artery of the retina perfuses the retina to the outer plexiform layer, and the choriocapillaris supplies the outer five layers of the retina. The Müller cells are radial glial cells that have support function. Myelin of the central nervous system (CNS) is produced by oligodendrocytes, which are not normally found in the retina. (Adapted with permission from Dudek RW: *High-Yield Histology.* Baltimore, Williams & Wilkins, 1997, p. 64.)

B. The **optic nerve** projects from the lamina cribrosa of the scleral canal, through the optic canal, to the optic chiasm (Figure 17-2).

    1. Transection causes ipsilateral blindness, with no direct pupillary light reflex.

    2. The section of the optic nerve at the optic chiasm transects all fibers from the ipsilateral retina as well as fibers from the contralateral inferior nasal quadrant that loop into the optic nerve. This **lesion** causes ipsilateral blindness and a contralateral upper temporal quadrant defect **(junction scotoma).**

C. The **optic chiasm** contains decussating fibers from the two nasal hemiretinas. It contains noncrossing fibers from the two temporal hemiretinas and projects fibers to the suprachiasmatic nucleus of the hypothalamus.

    1. Midsagittal transection or pressure (often from a pituitary tumor) causes bitemporal hemianopia.

    2. Bilateral lateral compression causes binasal hemianopia (calcified internal carotid arteries).

D. The **optic tract** contains fibers from the ipsilateral temporal hemiretina and the contralateral nasal hemiretina. It projects to the ipsilateral lateral geniculate body, pretectal nuclei, and superior colliculus. Transection causes contralateral hemianopia.

E. The **lateral geniculate body** is a six-layered nucleus. Layers 1, 4, and 6 receive crossed fibers; layers 2, 3, and 5 receive uncrossed fibers. The lateral geniculate body receives input from layer VI of the striate cortex (Brodmann's area 17). It also receives fibers from the ipsilateral temporal hemiretina and the contralateral nasal hemiretina. It projects through the geniculocalcarine tract to layer IV of the primary visual cortex (Brodmann's area 17).

F. The **geniculocalcarine tract (visual radiation)** projects through two divisions to the visual cortex.

    1. The **upper division** (Figure 17-3) projects to the upper bank of the calcarine sulcus, the cuneus. It contains input from the superior retinal quadrants, which represent the inferior visual field quadrants.

        a. Transection causes a contralateral lower quadrantanopia.

        b. Lesions that involve both cunei cause a lower altitudinal hemianopia (altitudinopia).

    2. The **lower division** (see Figure 17-3) loops from the lateral geniculate body anteriorly (Meyer's loop), then posteriorly, to terminate in the lower bank of the calcarine sulcus, the lingual gyrus. It contains input from the inferior retinal quadrants, which represent the superior visual field quadrants.

        a. Transection causes a **contralateral upper quadrantanopia** ("pie in the sky").

        b. Transection of both lingual gyri causes an **upper altitudinal hemianopia (altitudinopia).**

G. The **visual cortex (Brodmann's area 17)** is located on the banks of the calcarine fissure. The **cuneus** is the upper bank. The **lingual gyrus** is the lower bank. Lesions cause **contralateral hemianopia** with macular sparing. The visual cortex has a **retinotopic organization:**

    1. The **posterior area** receives macular input (central vision).

    2. The **intermediate area** receives paramacular input (peripheral input).

    3. The **anterior area** receives monocular input.

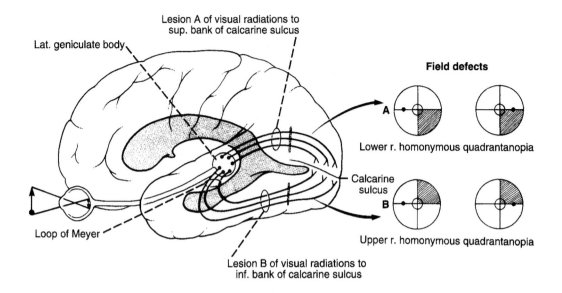

Figure 17-3.   Relations of the left upper and left lower divisions of the geniculocalcarine tract to the lateral ventricle and calcarine sulcus. Transection of the upper division (A) results in right lower homonymous quadrantanopia. Transection of the lower division (B) results in right upper homonymous quadrantanopia. (Reprinted with permission from Fix JD: *BRS Neuroanatomy.* Baltimore, Williams & Wilkins, 1997, p. 261.)

III. THE PUPILLARY LIGHT REFLEX PATHWAY (Figure 17-4) has an afferent limb (CN II) and an efferent limb (CN III). It includes the following structures:

    A. Ganglion cells of the retina, which project bilaterally to the pretectal nuclei

    B. The pretectal nucleus of the midbrain, which projects (through the posterior commissure) crossed and uncrossed fibers to the Edinger-Westphal nucleus

    C. The Edinger-Westphal nucleus of CN III, which gives rise to preganglionic parasympathetic fibers. These fibers exit the midbrain with CN III and synapse with postganglionic parasympathetic neurons of the ciliary ganglion.

    D. The ciliary ganglion, which gives rise to postganglionic parasympathetic fibers. These fibers innervate the sphincter muscle of the iris.

IV. THE PUPILLARY DILATION PATHWAY (Figure 17-5) is mediated by the sympathetic division of the autonomic nervous system. Interruption of this pathway at any level causes ipsilateral Horner's syndrome. It includes the following structures:

    A. The hypothalamus. Hypothalamic neurons of the paraventricular nucleus project directly to the ciliospinal center (T1–T2) of the intermediolateral cell column of the spinal cord.

    B. The ciliospinal center of Budge (T1–T2) projects preganglionic sympathetic fibers through the sympathetic trunk to the superior cervical ganglion.

    C. The superior cervical ganglion projects postganglionic sympathetic fibers through the perivascular plexus of the carotid system to the dilator muscle of the iris. Postganglionic sympathetic fibers pass through the **tympanic cavity** and **cavernous sinus** and enter the orbit through the **superior orbital fissure.**

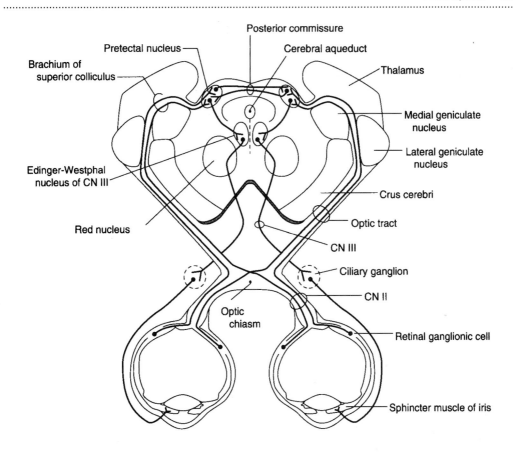

Figure 17-4. The pupillary light pathway. Light shined into one eye causes both pupils to constrict. The response in the stimulated eye is called the direct pupillary light reflex. The response in the opposite eye is called the consensual pupillary light reflex. *CN* = cranial nerve.

V. THE NEAR REFLEX AND ACCOMMODATION PATHWAY

  A. The **cortical visual pathway** projects from the primary visual cortex (Brodmann's area 17) to the visual association cortex (Brodmann's area 19).

  B. The **visual association cortex (Brodmann's area 19)** projects through the corticotectal tract to the superior colliculus and pretectal nucleus.

  C. The **superior colliculus** and **pretectal nucleus** project to the **oculomotor complex** of the **midbrain.** This complex includes the following structures:

  1. The **rostral Edinger-Westphal nucleus,** which mediates pupillary constriction through the ciliary ganglion

  2. The **caudal Edinger-Westphal nucleus,** which mediates contraction of the ciliary muscle. This contraction increases the refractive power of the lens.

  3. The **medial rectus subnucleus of CN III,** which mediates convergence

VI. CORTICAL AND SUBCORTICAL CENTERS FOR OCULAR MOTILITY

  A. The **frontal eye field** is located in the posterior part of the middle frontal gyrus (Brodmann's area 8). It regulates voluntary (saccadic) eye movements.

Figure 17-5. Ocular motor palsies and pupillary syndromes. (*A*) Relative afferent (Marcus Gunn) pupil, left eye. (*B*) Horner's syndrome, left eye. (*C*) Internuclear ophthalmoplegia, right eye. (*D*) Third-nerve palsy, left eye. (*E*) Sixth-nerve palsy, right eye. (*F*) Paralysis of upward gaze and convergence (Parinaud's syndrome). (*G*) Fourth-nerve palsy, right eye. (*H*) Argyll Robertson pupil. (*I*) Destructive lesion of the right frontal eye field. (*J*) Third-nerve palsy with ptosis, right eye.

1. **Stimulation** (e.g., from an irritative lesion) causes **contralateral deviation of the eyes** (i.e., away from the lesion).

2. **Destruction** causes **transient ipsilateral conjugate deviation of the eyes** (i.e., toward the lesion).

B. Occipital eye fields are located in Brodmann's areas 18 and 19 of the occipital lobes. These fields are cortical centers for involuntary (smooth) pursuit and tracking movements. **Stimulation** causes contralateral conjugate deviation of the eyes.

C. The **subcortical center for lateral conjugate gaze** is located in the abducent nucleus of the pons (Figure 17-6). Some authorities place the "center" in the paramedian pontine reticular formation.

1. It receives input from the contralateral frontal eye field.

2. It projects to the ipsilateral lateral rectus muscle and through the medial longitudinal fasciculus (MLF) to the contralateral medial rectus subnucleus of the oculomotor complex.

D. The **subcortical center for vertical conjugate gaze** is located in the midbrain at the level of the posterior commissure. It is called the rostral interstitial nucleus of the MLF and is associated with **Parinaud's syndrome** (see Figures 14-3A and 17-5F).

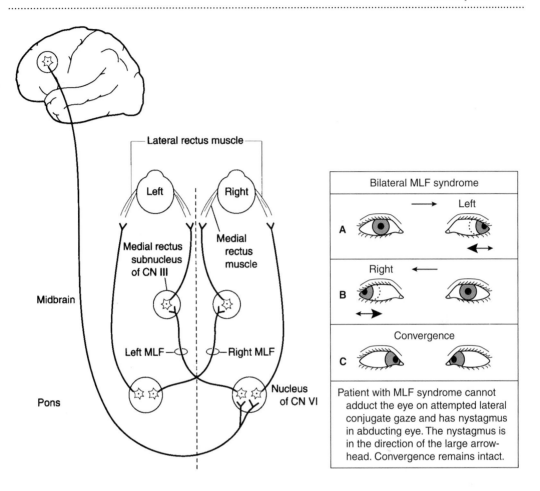

Figure 17-6.   Connections of the pontine center for lateral conjugate gaze. Lesions of the medial longitudinal fasciculus (*MLF*) between the abducent and oculomotor nuclei result in medial rectus palsy on attempted lateral conjugate gaze and horizontal nystagmus in the abducting eye. Convergence remains intact (*inset*). A unilateral MLF lesion would affect only the ipsilateral medial rectus. CN = cranial nerve.

VII. CLINICAL CORRELATION

A. In **MLF syndrome,** or **internuclear ophthalmoplegia** (see Figure 17-5), there is damage (demyelination) to the MLF between the abducent and oculomotor nuclei. It causes **medial rectus palsy on attempted lateral conjugate gaze** and monocular horizontal nystagmus in the abducting eye. **(Convergence is normal.)** This syndrome is most commonly seen in **multiple sclerosis.**

B. **One-and-a-half syndrome** consists of bilateral lesions of the MLF and a unilateral lesion of the abducent nucleus. On attempted lateral conjugate gaze, the only muscle that functions is the intact lateral rectus.

C. **Argyll Robertson pupil** (pupillary light–near dissociation) is the absence of a miotic reaction to light, both direct and consensual, with the preservation of a miotic reaction to near stimulus (accommodation–convergence). It occurs in **syphilis** and **diabetes.**

D. Horner's syndrome is caused by transection of the oculosympathetic pathway at any level (see IV). This syndrome consists of miosis, ptosis, apparent enophthalmos, and hemianhidrosis.

E. Relative afferent (Marcus Gunn) pupil results from a lesion of the optic nerve, the afferent limb of the pupillary light reflex (e.g., retrobulbar neuritis seen in multiple sclerosis). The diagnosis can be made with the swinging flashlight test (see Figure 17-5A).

F. Transentorial (uncal) herniation occurs as a result of **increased supratentorial pressure,** which is commonly caused by a brain tumor or hematoma (subdural or epidural).

   1. The pressure cone forces the parahippocampal uncus through the tentorial incisure.

   2. The impacted uncus forces the contralateral crus cerebri against the tentorial edge (Kernohan's notch) and puts pressure on the ipsilateral CN III and posterior cerebral artery. As a result, the following neurologic defects occur.

      a. Ipsilateral hemiparesis occurs as a result of pressure on the corticospinal tract, which is located in the contralateral crus cerebri.

      b. A **fixed and dilated pupil, ptosis,** and a **"down-and-out" eye** are caused by pressure on the ipsilateral oculomotor nerve.

      c. Contralateral homonymous hemianopia is caused by compression of the posterior cerebral artery, which irrigates the visual cortex.

G. Papilledema (choked disk) is noninflammatory congestion of the optic disk as a result of increased intracranial pressure. It is most commonly caused by brain tumors, subdural hematoma, or hydrocephalus. It usually **does not alter visual acuity,** but it may cause bilateral **enlarged blind spots.** It is often asymmetric and is greater on the side of the supratentorial lesion.

H. Adie's pupil is a large tonic that reacts slowly to light but does react to near (light-near dissociation). Frequently seen in females with absent knee or ankle jerks.

18

Autonomic Nervous System

I. INTRODUCTION. The autonomic nervous system (ANS) is a general visceral efferent motor system that **controls and regulates smooth muscle, cardiac muscle, and glands.**

 A. The ANS consists of two types of **projection neurons:**

 1. Preganglionic neurons

 2. Postganglionic neurons. Sympathetic ganglia have interneurons.

 B. **Autonomic output** is controlled by the **hypothalamus.**

 C. The ANS has **three divisions:**

 1. **Sympathetic.** Figure 18-1 shows the sympathetic innervation of the ANS.

 2. **Parasympathetic.** Figure 18-2 shows the parasympathetic innervation of the ANS. Table 18-1 compares the effects of sympathetic and parasympathetic activity on organ systems.

 3. **Enteric.** The enteric division includes the intramural ganglia of the gastrointestinal tract, submucosal plexus, and myenteric plexus.

II. CRANIAL NERVES (CN) WITH PARASYMPATHETIC COMPONENTS include the following:

 A. **CN III** (ciliary ganglion)

 B. **CN VII** (pterygopalatine and submandibular ganglia)

 C. **CN IX** (otic ganglion)

 D. **CN X** [terminal (mural) ganglia]

III. COMMUNICATING RAMI of the ANS include:

 A. **White communicating rami,** which are found between T-1 and L-3, are myelinated.

 B. **Gray communicating rami,** which are found at all spinal levels, are unmyelinated.

IV. NEUROTRANSMITTERS of the ANS include:

 A. **Acetylcholine,** which is the neurotransmitter of the preganglionic neurons

 B. **Norepinephrine,** which is the neurotransmitter of the postganglionic neurons, with the exception of sweat glands and some blood vessels that receive cholinergic sympathetic innervation

 C. **Dopamine,** which is the neurotransmitter of the small intensely fluorescent (SIF) cells, which are interneurons of the sympathetic ganglia

Figure 18-1. The sympathetic (thoracolumbar) innervation of the autonomic nervous system. The entire sympathetic innervation of the head is through the superior cervical ganglion. Gray communicating rami are found at all spinal cord levels. White communicating rami are found only in spinal segments T-1 through L-3.

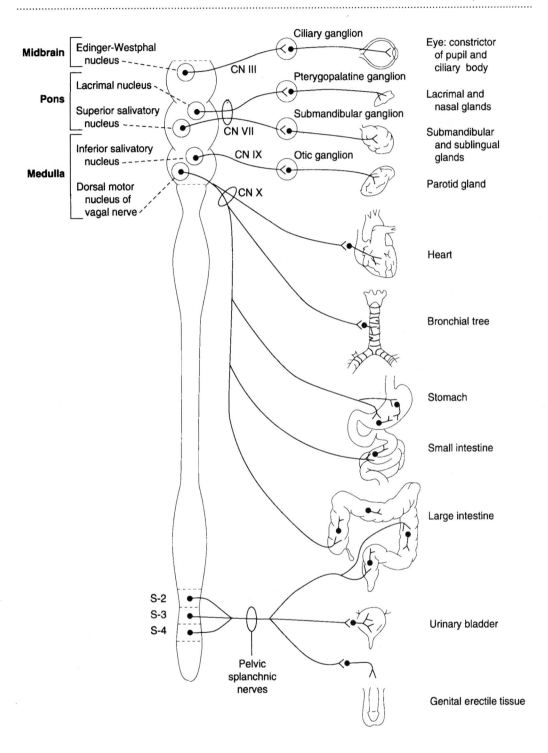

Figure 18-2. The parasympathetic (craniosacral) innervation of the autonomic nervous system. Sacral outflow includes segments S-2 through S-4. Cranial outflow is mediated through cranial nerves (CN) III, VII, IX, and X.

Table 18-1
Sympathetic and Parasympathetic Activity on Organ Systems

Structure	Sympathetic Function	Parasympathetic Function
Eye		
Radial muscle of iris	Dilation of pupil (mydriasis)	
Circular muscle of iris		Constriction of pupil (miosis)
Ciliary muscle of ciliary body		Contraction for near vision
Lacrimal gland		Stimulation of secretion
Salivary glands	Viscous secretion	Watery secretion
Sweat glands		
Thermoregulatory	Increase	
Apocrine (stress)	Increase	
Heart		
Sinoatrial node	Acceleration	Deceleration (vagal arrest)
Atrioventricular node	Increase in conduction velocity	Decrease in conduction velocity
Contractility	Increase	Decrease (atria)
Vascular smooth muscle		
Skin, splanchnic vessels	Contraction	
Skeletal muscle vessels	Relaxation	
Bronchiolar smooth muscle	Relaxation	Contraction
Gastrointestinal tract		
Smooth muscle		
Walls	Relaxation	Contraction
Sphincters	Contraction	Relaxation
Secretion and motility	Decrease	Increase
Genitourinary tract		
Smooth muscle		
Bladder wall	Little or no effect	Contraction
Sphincter	Contraction	Relaxation
Penis, seminal vesicles	Ejaculation*	Erection*
Adrenal medulla	Secretion of epinephrine and norepinephrine	
Metabolic functions		
Liver	Gluconeogenesis and glycogenolysis	
Fat cells	Lipolysis	
Kidney	Renin release	

*Note erection versus ejaculation: Remember **p**oint and **s**hoot: p = parasympathetic, s = sympathetic.
(Reprinted with permission from Fix J: *BRS Neuroanatomy*. Media, PA, Williams & Wilkins, 1991.)

    D. Vasoactive intestinal polypeptide (VIP), a vasodilator that is colocalized with acetylcholine in some postganglionic parasympathetic fibers

    E. Nitric oxide (NO), a newly discovered neurotransmitter that is responsible for the relaxation of smooth muscle. It is also responsible for penile erection (see Chapter 22).

V. CLINICAL CORRELATION

    A. Megacolon (Hirschsprung's disease, or congenital aganglionic megacolon) is characterized by extreme dilation and hypertrophy of the colon, with fecal retention, and by the absence of ganglion cells in the myenteric plexus. It occurs when neural crest cells do not migrate into the colon.

    B. Familial dysautonomia (Riley-Day syndrome) predominantly affects Jewish children. It is an autosomal recessive trait that is characterized by abnormal sweating, unstable blood pressure (e.g., orthostatic hypotension), difficulty in feeding (as a result of inadequate muscle tone in the gastrointestinal tract), and progressive sensory loss. It results in the loss of neurons in the autonomic and sensory ganglia.

C. **Raynaud's disease** is a painful disorder of the terminal arteries of the extremities. It is characterized by idiopathic paroxysmal bilateral cyanosis of the digits (as a result of arterial and arteriolar constriction because of cold or emotion). It may be treated by preganglionic sympathectomy.

D. **Peptic ulcer disease** results from excessive production of hydrochloric acid because of increased parasympathetic (tone) stimulation.

E. **Horner's syndrome** (see Chapter 17) is oculosympathetic paralysis.

F. **Shy-Drager syndrome** involves preganglionic sympathetic neurons from the intermediolateral cell column. It is characterized by orthostatic hypotension, anhidrosis, impotence, and bladder atonicity.

G. **Botulism.** The toxin of *Clostridium botulinum* blocks the release of acetylcholine and results in paralysis of all striated muscles. Autonomic effects include dry eyes, dry mouth, and gastrointestinal ileus (bowel obstruction).

H. **Lambert-Eaton myasthenic syndrome** (see Chapter 22)

19
Hypothalamus

I. INTRODUCTION

A. **General structure and function.** The hypothalamus is a **division of the diencephalon** that subserves three systems: the autonomic nervous system, endocrine system, and limbic system. The hypothalamus helps to maintain homeostasis.

B. **Major hypothalamic nuclei and their functions**

1. The **medial preoptic nucleus** (Figure 19-1) regulates the release of gonadotropic hormones from the adenohypophysis. It contains the sexually dimorphic nucleus, the development of which depends on testosterone levels.

2. The **suprachiasmatic nucleus** receives direct input from the retina. It plays a role in the regulation of circadian rhythms.

Paraventricular and supraoptic nuclei
• regulate water balance
• produce ADH and oxytocin
• destruction causes diabetes insipidus
• paraventricular nucleus projects to autonomic nuclei of brain stem and spinal cord

Anterior nucleus
• thermal regulation (dissipation of heat)
• stimulates parasympathetic NS
• destruction results in hyperthermia

Preoptic area
• contains sexual dimorphic nucleus
• regulates release of gonadotropic hormones

Suprachiasmatic nucleus
• receives input from retina
• controls circadian rhythms

Dorsomedial nucleus
• stimulation results in obesity and savage behavior

Posterior nucleus
• thermal regulation (conservation of heat)
• destruction results in inability to thermoregulate
• stimulates the sympathetic NS

Lateral nucleus
• stimulation induces eating
• destruction results in starvation

Mamillary body
• receives input from hippocampal formation via fornix
• projects to anterior nucleus of thalamus
• contains hemorrhagic lesions in Wernicke's encephalopathy

Ventromedial nucleus
• satiety center
• destruction results in obesity and savage behavior

Midbrain

CN III

Pons

Arcuate nucleus
• produces hypothalamic releasing factors
• contains DOPA-ergic neurons that inhibit prolactin release

Figure 19-1. Major hypothalamic nuclei and their functions. *ADH* = antidiuretic hormone; *CN* = cranial nerve; *DOPA* = dopamine; *NS* = nervous system.

3. The **anterior nucleus** plays a role in temperature regulation. It stimulates the parasympathetic nervous system. Destruction results in hyperthermia.

4. The **paraventricular nucleus** (Figure 19-2) synthesizes antidiuretic hormone (ADH), oxytocin, and corticotropin-releasing hormone. It gives rise to the supra-opticohypophyseal tract, which projects to the neurohypophysis. It regulates water balance (conservation) and projects directly to the autonomic nuclei of the brain stem and all levels of the spinal cord. Destruction results in diabetes insipidus.

5. The **supraoptic nucleus** synthesizes ADH and oxytocin (similar to the paraventricular nucleus).

6. The **dorsomedial nucleus.** In animals, savage behavior results when this nucleus is stimulated.

7. The **ventromedial nucleus** is considered a satiety center. When stimulated, it inhibits the urge to eat. Bilateral destruction results in hyperphagia, obesity, and savage behavior.

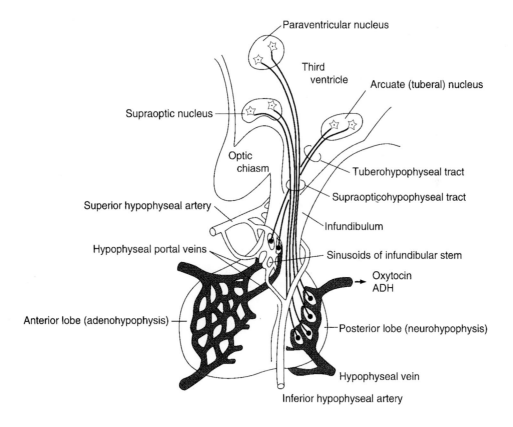

Figure 19-2.   The hypophyseal portal system. The paraventricular and supraoptic nuclei produce antidiuretic hormone (*ADH*) and oxytocin and transport them through the supraopticohypophyseal tract to the capillary bed of the neurohypophysis. The arcuate nucleus of the infundibulum transports hypothalamic-stimulating hormones through the tuberohypophyseal tract to the sinusoids of the infundibular stem. These sinusoids then drain into the secondary capillary plexus in the adenohypophysis.

8. The **arcuate (infundibular) nucleus** contains neurons that produce factors that stimulate or inhibit the action of the hypothalamus. This nucleus gives rise to the tuberohypophyseal tract, which terminates in the hypophyseal portal system (see Figure 19-2) of the infundibulum (medium eminence). It contains neurons that produce dopamine (i.e., prolactin-inhibiting factor).

9. The **mamillary nucleus** receives input from the hippocampal formation through the postcommissural fornix. It projects to the anterior nucleus of the thalamus through the mamillothalamic tract (part of the Papez circuit). Patients with Wernicke's encephalopathy, which is a thiamine (vitamin B_1) deficiency, have lesions in the mamillary nucleus. Lesions are also associated with alcoholism.

10. The **posterior hypothalamic nucleus** plays a role in thermal regulation (i.e., conservation and increased production of heat). Lesions result in **poikilothermia** (i.e., inability to thermoregulate).

11. The **lateral hypothalamic nucleus** induces eating when stimulated. **Lesions** cause **anorexia** and **starvation.**

C. Major fiber systems of the hypothalamus

1. The **fornix** is the largest projection to the hypothalamus. It projects from the hippocampal formation to the mamillary nucleus, anterior nucleus of the thalamus, and septal area. The fornix then projects from the septal area to the hippocampal formation.

2. The **medial forebrain bundle** traverses the entire lateral hypothalamic area. It interconnects the orbitofrontal cortex, septal area, hypothalamus, and midbrain.

3. The **mamillothalamic tract** projects from the mamillary nuclei to the anterior nucleus of the thalamus (part of the Papez circuit).

4. The **stria terminalis** is the major pathway from the amygdala. It interconnects the septal area, hypothalamus, and amygdala.

5. The **supraopticohypophysial tract** conducts fibers from the supraoptic and paraventricular nuclei to the neurohypophysis, which is the release site for ADH and oxytocin.

6. The **tuberohypophysial (tuberoinfundibular) tract** conducts fibers from the arcuate nucleus to the hypophyseal portal system (see Figure 19-2).

7. The **hypothalamospinal tract** contains direct descending autonomic fibers. These fibers influence the preganglionic sympathetic neurons of the intermediolateral cell column and preganglionic neurons of the sacral parasympathetic nucleus. Interruption above the first thoracic segment (T-1) causes Horner's syndrome.

II. FUNCTIONS

A. Autonomic function

1. The **anterior hypothalamus** has an excitatory effect on the parasympathetic nervous system.

2. The **posterior hypothalamus** has an excitatory effect on the sympathetic nervous system.

B. Temperature regulation

1. The **anterior hypothalamus** regulates and maintains body temperature. Destruction causes hyperthermia.

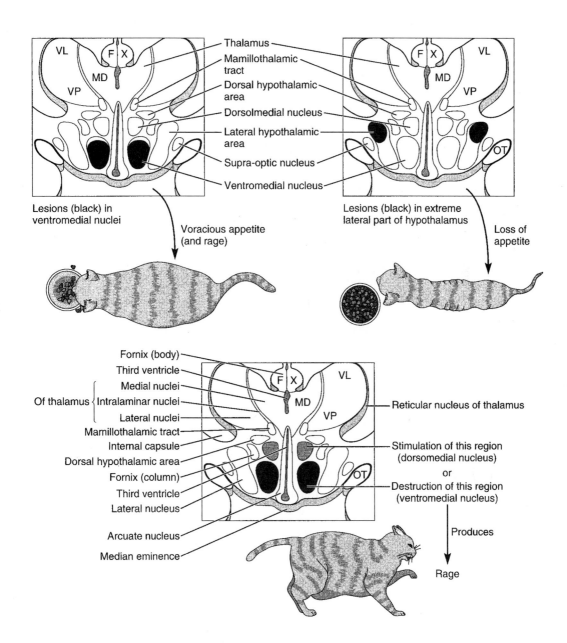

Figure 19-3.   Coronal section through the hypothalamus at the level of the dorsomedial, vetromedial, and lateral hypothalamus nuclei. Lesions or stimulation of these nuclei result in obesity, cachexia, and rage. The column of the fornix separates the medial from the lateral hypothalamic zones. A lesion of the OT results in a contralateral hemianopia. FX = fornix; MD = medial dorsal nucleus of thalamus; OT = optic tract; VL = ventral lateral nucleus of thalamus; VP = ventral posterior nucleus of thalamus. (Reprinted with permission from Fix JD: *BRS Neuroanatomy*, 3rd ed. Baltimore, Williams & Wilkins, 1996, p. 313.)

2. The **posterior hypothalamus** helps to produce and conserve heat. Destruction causes the inability to thermoregulate.

C. Water balance regulation. The **paraventricular nucleus** synthesizes ADH, which controls water excretion by the kidneys.

D. Food intake regulation. Two hypothalamic nuclei play a role in the control of appetite.

1. When stimulated, the **ventromedial nucleus** inhibits the urge to eat. Bilateral destruction results in hyperphagia, obesity, and savage behavior.

2. When stimulated, the **lateral hypothalamic nucleus** induces the urge to eat. Destruction causes starvation and emaciation.

III. CLINICAL CORRELATION

A. Diabetes insipidus, which is characterized by polyuria and polydipsia, is the best known hypothalamic syndrome. It results from lesions of the ADH pathways to the posterior lobe of the pituitary gland.

B. The **syndrome of inappropriate ADH secretion** is usually caused by lung tumors or drug therapy (e.g., carbamazepine, chlorpromazine).

C. Craniopharyngioma is a congenital tumor that originates from remnants of Rathke's pouch (see Chapter 4). This tumor is usually calcified. It is the most common supratentorial tumor in children and the most common cause of hypopituitarism in children.

1. Pressure on the chiasma results in bitemporal hemianopia.

2. Pressure on the hypothalamus causes hypothalamic syndrome (i.e., adiposity, diabetes insipidus, disturbance of temperature regulation, and somnolence).

D. Pituitary adenomas account for 15% of clinical symptomatic intracranial tumors. They are rarely seen in children. When pituitary adenomas are endocrine-active, they cause endocrine abnormalities (e.g., amenorrhea and galactorrhea from a prolactin-secreting adenoma, the most common type).

1. Pressure on the chiasma results in bitemporal hemianopia.

2. Pressure on the hypothalamus may cause hypothalamus syndrome (Figure 19-3).

20

Limbic System

I. INTRODUCTION. The limbic system is considered the anatomic substrate that underlies behavioral and emotional expression. It is expressed through the hypothalamus by way of the autonomic nervous system.

II. MAJOR COMPONENTS AND CONNECTIONS

A. The **orbitofrontal cortex** mediates the conscious perception of smell. It has reciprocal connections with the mediodorsal nucleus of the thalamus. It is interconnected through the medial forebrain bundle with the septal area and hypothalamic nuclei.

B. The **mediodorsal nucleus of the thalamus** has reciprocal connections with the orbitofrontal and prefrontal cortices as well as the hypothalamus. It receives input from the amygdala and plays a role in affective behavior and memory.

C. The **anterior nucleus of the thalamus** receives input from the mamillary nucleus through the mamillothalamic tract and fornix. It projects to the cingulate gyrus and is a major link in the Papez circuit.

D. The **septal area** is a telencephalic structure. It has reciprocal connections with the hippocampal formation through the fornix and with the hypothalamus through the medial forebrain bundle. It projects through the stria medullaris (thalami) to the habenular nucleus.

E. The **limbic lobe** includes the subcallosal area, paraterminal gyrus, cingulate gyrus and isthmus, and parahippocampal gyrus, which includes the uncus. It contains, buried in the parahippocampal gyrus, the hippocampal formation and amygdaloid nuclear complex.

F. The **hippocampal formation** is a sheet of archicortex that is jelly-rolled into the parahippocampal gyrus. It functions in learning, memory, and recognition of novelty. It receives major input through the entorhinal cortex and projects major output through the fornix. Its **major structures include the following:**

1. The **dentate gyrus,** which has a three-layered archicortex. It contains granule cells that receive hippocampal input and project output to the pyramidal cells of the hippocampus and subiculum.

2. The **hippocampus (cornu Ammonis),** which has a three-layered archicortex. It contains pyramidal cells that project through the fornix to the septal area and hypothalamus.

3. The **subiculum,** which receives input through the hippocampal pyramidal cells. It projects through the fornix to the mamillary nuclei and the anterior nucleus of the thalamus.

G. The **amygdaloid complex (amygdala)** [Figure 20-1; see also Figure 21-1] is a basal ganglion that underlies the parahippocampal uncus. In humans, stimulation causes fear and signs of sympathetic overactivity. In other animals, stimulation results in cessation of activity and heightened attentiveness. Lesions cause placidity and hypersexual behavior.

1. Input is from the sensory association cortices, olfactory bulb and cortex, hypothalamus and septal area, and hippocampal formation.

2. Output is through the stria terminalis to the hypothalamus and septal area. There is also output to the mediodorsal nucleus of the thalamus.

H. The **hypothalamus** has reciprocal connections with the amygdala.

I. The **limbic midbrain nuclei** and **associated neurotransmitters** include the ventral tegmental area (dopamine), raphe nuclei (serotonin), and locus ceruleus (norepinephrine).

III. THE PAPEZ CIRCUIT (Figure 20-2) includes the following limbic structures:

A. The **hippocampal formation,** which projects through the fornix to the mamillary nucleus and septal area

B. The **mamillary nucleus**

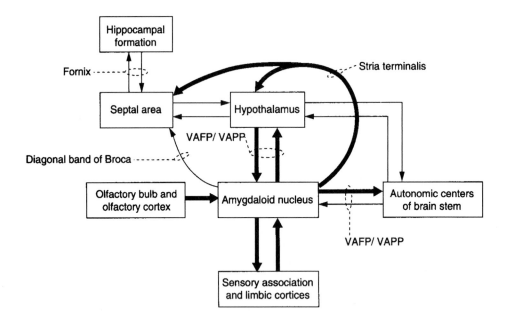

Figure 20-1. Major connections of the amygdaloid nucleus. This nucleus receives input from three major sources: the olfactory system, sensory association and limbic cortices, and hypothalamus. Major output is through two channels: the stria terminalis projects to the hypothalamus and the septal area, and the ventral amygdalofugal pathway (*VAFP*) projects to the hypothalamus, brain stem, and spinal cord. A smaller efferent bundle, the diagonal band of Broca, projects to the septal area. Afferent fibers from the hypothalamus and brain stem enter the amygdaloid nucleus through the ventral amygdalopetal pathway (*VAPP*).

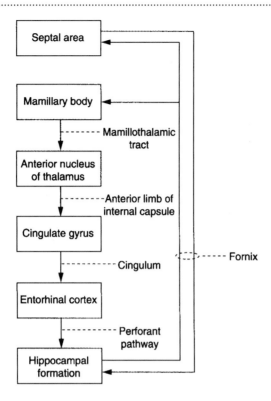

Figure 20-2. Major afferent and efferent limbic connections of the hippocampal formation. This formation has three components: the hippocampus (cornu Ammonis), subiculum, and dentate gyrus. The hippocampus projects to the septal area, the subiculum projects to the mamillary nuclei, and the dentate gyrus does not project beyond the hippocampal formation. The circuit of Papez follows this route: hippocampal formation to mamillary nucleus to anterior thalamic nucleus to cingulate gyrus to entorhinal cortex to hippocampal formation.

  C. The **anterior thalamic nucleus**

  D. The **cingulate gyrus** (Brodmann's areas 23 and 24)

  E. The **entorhinal area** (Brodmann's area 28)

IV. CLINICAL CORRELATION

  A. Klüver-Bucy syndrome results from bilateral ablation of the anterior temporal lobes, including the amygdaloid nuclei. It causes psychic blindness (visual agnosia), hyperphagia, docility (placidity), and hypersexuality.

  B. Amnestic (confabulatory) syndrome results from bilateral infarction of the hippocampal formation (i.e., hippocampal branches of the posterior cerebral arteries and anterior choroidal arteries of the internal carotid arteries). It causes anterograde amnesia (i.e., inability to learn and retain new information). **Memory loss suggests hippocampal pathology.**

  C. Foster Kennedy syndrome results from **meningioma** of the **olfactory groove.** The meningioma compresses the olfactory tract and optic nerve. Ipsilateral anosmia and

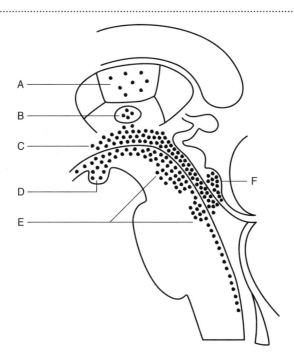

Figure 20-3.   Midsagittal section through the brain stem and diencephalon showing the distribution of lesions in Wernicke's encephalopathy. (A) Mediodorsal nucleus of the thalamus. (B) Massa intermedia. (C) Periventricular area. (D) Mamillary nuclei. (E) Midbrain and pontine tegmentum. (F) Inferior colliculus. Lesions in the mamillary nuclei are associated with Wernicke's encephalopathy and thiamine (vitamin B$_1$) deficiency.

    optic atrophy and contralateral papilledema occur as a result of increased intracranial pressure.

   D. The **hippocampus** is the most epileptogenic part of the cerebrum. Lesions may cause psychomotor attacks. Sommer's sector is very sensitive to ischemia.

   E. Bilateral transection of the fornix may cause the acute amnestic syndrome (i.e., inability to consolidate short-term memory into long-term memory).

   F. **Wernicke's encephalopathy** results from a thiamine (vitamin B$_1$) deficiency. The clinical triad includes ocular disturbances and nystagmus, gait ataxia, and mental dysfunction. Pathologic features include mamillary nuclei, MD nuclei of the thalamus, and periaqueductal gray and pontine tegmentum (Figure 20-3).

   G. **Strachan's syndrome** results from high-dose thiamine (vitamin B$_1$) therapy. The clinical triad includes spinal ataxia, optic atrophy, and nerve deafness.

   H. Bilateral destruction or removal of the cingulate gyri causes loss of initiative and inhibition as well as dulling of the emotions. Memory is unaffected. Lesions of the anterior cingulate gyri cause placidity. Cingulectomy is used to treat severe anxiety and depression (Figure 20-4).

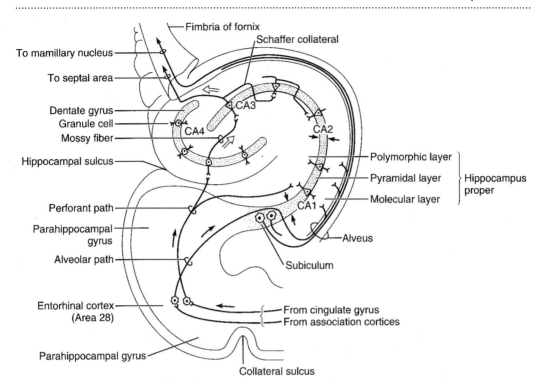

Figure 20-4. Major connections of the hippocampal formation. The hippocampal formation (HF) consists of three parts: hippocampus, dentate gyrus, and subiculum. The two major hypothalamic output pathways are: (*1*) granule cell via mossy fiber to pyramidal cell via precommissural fornix to septal nuclei, and (*2*) subicular neuron via postcommissural fornix to the medial mamillary nucleus. The HF plays an important role in learning and memory, and lesions of the HF result in short-term memory defects. In Alzheimer disease, loss of cells in the HF and entorhinal cortex leads to loss of memory and cognitive function. CA = cornu ammonis. The sector CA1 is very sensitive to hypoxia (cardiac arrest or stroke). (Reprinted with permission from Fix JD: *BRS Neuroanatomy*, 3rd ed. Baltimore, Williams & Wilkins, 1996, p. 332.)

21

Basal Ganglia and Striatal Motor System

I. BASAL GANGLIA (Figure 21-1)

  A. Components

   1. Caudate nucleus

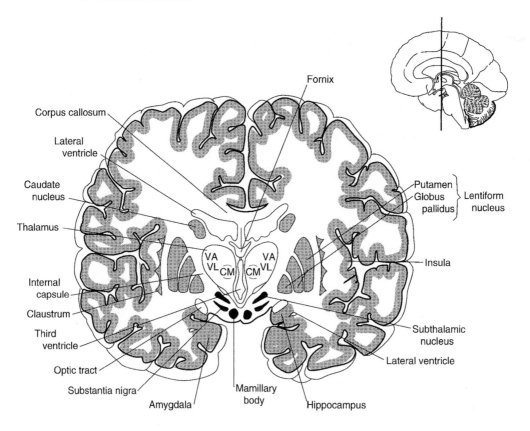

Figure 21-1.   Coronal section through the midthalamus at the level of the mamillary bodies. The basal ganglia are all prominent at this level and include the striatum and lentiform nucleus. The subthalamic nucleus and substantia nigra are important components of the striatal motor system. CM = centromedian nucleus; VA = ventral anterior nucleus; VL = ventral lateral nucleus. (Modified with permission from Woolsey TA, Hanaway J, Gado MH: *The Brain Atlas: A Visual Guide to the Human Central Nervous System*, 2nd ed. Hoboken, John Wiley & Sons, 2003, p. 68.)

2. Putamen

3. Globus pallidus

B. Grouping of the basal ganglia

1. The **striatum** consists of the caudate nucleus and putamen.

2. The **lentiform nucleus** consists of the globus pallidus and putamen.

3. The **corpus striatum** consists of the lentiform nucleus and caudate nucleus.

4. The **claustrum** lies between the lentiform nucleus and the insular cortex. It has reciprocal connections between the sensory cortices (i.e., visual cortex) [Figures 21-2, 21-3, and 21-4].

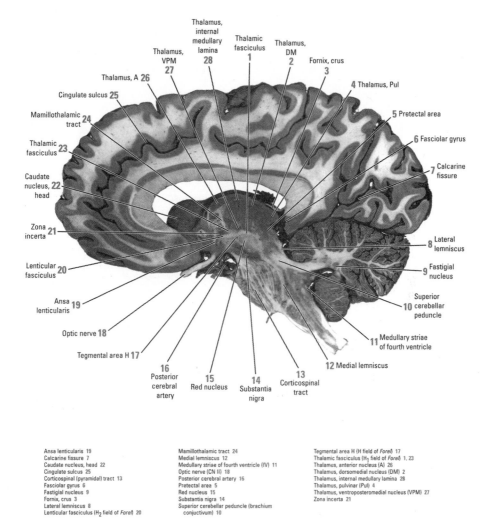

Ansa lenticularis 19
Calcarine fissure 7
Caudate nucleus, head 22
Cingulate sulcus 25
Corticospinal (pyramidal) tract 13
Fasciolar gyrus 6
Fastigial nucleus 9
Fornix, crus 3
Lateral lemniscus 8
Lenticular fasciculus (H₂ field of *Forel*) 20

Mamillothalamic tract 24
Medial lemniscus 12
Medullary striae of fourth ventricle (IV) 11
Optic nerve (CN II) 18
Posterior cerebral artery 16
Pretectal area 5
Red nucleus 15
Substantia nigra 14
Superior cerebellar peduncle (brachium conjuctivum) 10

Tegmental area H (H field of *Forel*) 17
Thalamic fasciculus (H₁ field of *Forel*) 1, 23
Thalamus, anterior nucleus (A) 26
Thalamus, dorsomedial nucleus (DM) 2
Thalamus, internal medullary lamina 28
Thalamus, pulvinar (Pul) 4
Thalamus, ventroposteromedial nucleus (VPM) 27
Zona incerta 21

Figure 21-2. A parasagittal section through the caudate nucleus (5) and the substantia nigra (10): subthalamic nucleus (11), internal capsule (12), thalamus (13), cingulate gyrus (14). (Modified with permission from Woolsey TA, Hanaway J, Gado MH: *The Brain Atlas: A Visual Guide to the Human Central Nervous System,* 2nd ed. Hoboken, John Wiley & Sons, 2003, p. 128.)

Hypothalamus,
lateral preoptic
nucleus
29

Fornix,
column
30

Cingulate
gyrus
1

Internal capsule, anterior limb **28**

Globus pallidus, medial **27**
medullary lamina

Globus pallidus, GPe **26**

Insula, short gyri **25**

Globus pallidus, GPi **24**

Insula, long gyrus **23**

Internal capsule, **22**
posterior limb

Middle cerebral **21**
artery, branch

Internal capsule, **20**
retrolenticular part

Thalamo-occipital **19**
fasciculus

Choroid plexus of lateral ventricle **18**

Thalamus, Pul **17**

16
Great
cerebral vein

15
Longitudinal
cerebral fissure

14
Stria medullaris
of thalamus

2 Anterior commissure

3 Caudate nucleus, head

4 Putamen

5 Lateral sulcus

Hypothalamus,
6 paraventricular
nucleus

Globus pallidus,
7 lateral medullary
lamina

8 Temporal
operculum

9 Interthalamic
adhesion

10 Thalamus, VL

11 Thalamus, DM

12 Optic radiation

13 Hippocampus, tail

Anterior commissure **2**
Caudate nucleus, head **3**
Choroid plexus of lateral ventricle **18**
Cingulate gyrus **1**
Fornix, column **30**
Globus pallidus, external (lateral) segment (GPe) **26**
Globus pallidus, internal (medial) segment (GPi) **24**
Globus pallidus, lateral medullary lamina **7**
Globus pallidus, medial medullary lamina **27**
Great cerebral vein (vein of *Galen*) **16**

Hippocampus, tail **13**
Hypothalamus, lateral preoptic nucleus **29**
Hypothalamus, paraventricular nucleus **6**
Insula, long gyrus **23**
Insula, short gyri **25**
Internal capsule, anterior limb **28**
Internal capsule, posterior limb **22**
Internal capsule, retrolenticular part **20**
Interthalamic adhesion (massa intermedia) **9**
Lateral sulcus (*Sylvian* fissure) **5**

Longitudinal cerebral (interhemispheric) fissure **15**
Middle cerebral artery, branch **21**
Optic radiation **12**
Putamen **4**
Stria medullaris of thalamus **14**
Temporal operculum **8**
Thalamo-occipital fasciculus **19**
Thalamus, dorsomedial nucleus (DM) **11**
Thalamus, pulvinar (Pul) **17**
Thalamus, ventrolateral nucleus (VL) **10**

Figure 21-3.   An axial (horizontal) section through the anterior commissure (15) and the massa intermedia (16): internal capsule (6), globus pallidus (7), insular cortex (14), putamen (17), claustrum (2), head of caudate nucleus (18). (Modified with permission from Woolsey TA, Hanaway J, Gado MH: *The Brain Atlas: A Visual Guide to the Human Central Nervous System*, 2nd ed. Hoboken, John Wiley & Sons, 2003, p. 100.)

Anterior cerebral artery, pericallosal branch
26 Longitudinal cerebral fissure
1 Anterior cerebral artery, pericallosal branch
2 Corpus callosum, body
25 Septum pellucidum
3 Lateral septal nucleus
24 Superior occipitofrontal fasciculus
4 Caudate nucleus, head
23 Superior longitudinal fasciculus
5 Internal capsule, anterior limb
22 Globus pallidus, lateral medullary lamina
6 Globus pallidus, GPe
7 Insula
21 Middle cerebral artery
8 Lateral sulcus
20 Inferior occipitofrontal fasciculus
9 Uncinate fasciculus
19 Orbitofrontal fibers
10 Middle cerebral artery, lateral lenticulostriate branches
18 Anterior commissure
11 Anterior commissure, olfactory part
17 Amygdala
12 Anterior cerebral artery
16 Anterior perforated substance
15 Nucleus of diagonal band
14 Optic chiasm
13 Internal carotid artery

Amygdala 17
Anterior cerebral artery 12
Anterior cerebral artery, pericallosal branch 1
Anterior commissure 18
Anterior commissure, olfactory part 11
Anterior perforated substance 16
Caudate nucleus, head 4
Corpus callosum, body 2
Globus pallidus, external (lateral) segment (GPe) 6
Globus pallidus, lateral medullary lamina 22

Inferior occipitofrontal fasciculus 20
Insula 7
Internal capsule, anterior limb 5
Internal carotid artery 13
Lateral septal nucleus 3
Lateral sulcus (*Sylvian* fissure) 8
Longitudinal cerebral (interhemispheric) fissure 26
Middle cerebral artery 21
Middle cerebral artery, lateral lenticulostriate branches [medial lenticulostriate branches originate from the anterior cerebral artery] 10

Nucleus of diagonal band (diagonal band of *Broca*) 15
Optic chiasm 14
Orbitofrontal fibers 19
Septum pellucidum 25
Superior longitudinal fasciculus 23
Superior occipitofrontal fasciculus 24
Uncinate fasciculus 9

Figure 21-4. A coronal section through the lentiform nucleus and the amydaloid nucleus (1); the lentiform nucleus consists of the putamen (8) and the globus pallidus (7); the amygdaloid nucleus appears as a circular profile below the uncus. (Modified with permission from Woolsey TA, Hanaway J, Gado MH: *The Brain Atlas: A Visual Guide to the Human Central Nervous System*, 2nd ed. Hoboken, John Wiley & Sons, 2003, p. 60.)

II. THE STRIATAL (EXTRAPYRAMIDAL) MOTOR SYSTEM (see Figure 21-1) plays
a role in the initiation and execution of somatic motor activity, especially willed movement. It is also involved in automatic stereotyped postural and reflex motor activity (e.g.,
normal subjects swing their arms when they walk).

A. **Structure.** The striatal motor system includes the following structures:

1. **Neocortex**

2. **Striatum (caudatoputamen, or neostriatum)**

3. **Globus pallidus**

4. **Subthalamic nucleus**

5. **Substantia nigra** (i.e., pars compacta and pars reticularis)

6. **Thalamus** (ventral anterior, ventral lateral, and centromedian nuclei)

B. Figure 21-5 shows the **major afferent** and **efferent connections** of the striatal system.

C. **Neurotransmitters** (Figure 21-6)

III. CLINICAL CORRELATION

A. **Parkinson's disease** is a **degenerative disease** that affects the substantia nigra and
its projections to the striatum.

1. **Results.** Parkinson's disease causes a **depletion of dopamine** in the substantia

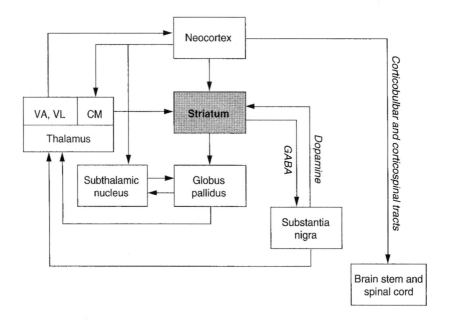

Figure 21-5. Major afferent and efferent connections of the striatal system. The striatum receives major
input from three sources: the thalamus, neocortex, and substantia nigra. The striatum projects to the globus
pallidus and substantia nigra. The globus pallidus is the effector nucleus of the striatal system; it projects to
the thalamus and subthalamic nucleus. The substantia nigra also projects to the thalamus. The striatal motor
system is expressed through the corticobulbar and corticospinal tracts. CM centromedian nucleus; GABA =
γ-aminobutyric acid; VA = ventral anterior nucleus; VL = ventral lateral nucleus.

Figure 21-6. Major neurotransmitters of the striatal motor system. Within the striatum, globus pallidus, and pars reticularis of the substantia nigra (*S. nigra*), γ-aminobutyric acid (*GABA*) is the predominant neurotransmitter. GABA may coexist in the same neuron with enkephalin (*ENK*) or substance P (*SP*). Dopamine-containing neurons are found in the pars compacta of the substantia nigra. Acetylcholine (*ACh*) is found in the local circuit neurons of the striatum. The subthalamic nucleus projects excitatory glutaminergic fibers to the globus pallidus. GLU = glutamate.

nigra and striatum as well as a **loss of melanin-containing dopaminergic neurons** in the substantia nigra.

2. **Clinical signs** are bradykinesia, stooped posture, shuffling gait, cogwheel rigidity, pill-rolling tremor, and masked facies. **Lewy bodies** are found in the melanin-containing neurons of the substantia nigra. **Progressive supranuclear palsy** is associated with Parkinson disease.

3. **Treatment** has been successful with L-Dopa. Surgical intervention includes **pallidotomy** (rigidity) and **ventral thalomotomy** (tremor).

B. **Methylphenyltetrahydropyridine (MPTP)-induced parkinsonism.** MPTP is an analog of meperidine (Demerol). It destroys dopaminergic neurons in the substantia nigra.

C. **Huntington's disease** (chorea) is an **inherited autosomal dominant movement disorder** that is traced to a single gene defect on chromosome 4.

1. It is associated with **degeneration of the cholinergic and γ-aminobutyric acid (GABA)-ergic neurons** of the striatum. It is accompanied by gyral atrophy in the frontal and temporal lobes.

2. **Glutamate excitotoxicity.** GLU is released in the striatum and binds to its receptors on striatal neurons resulting in an action potential. GLU is removed from the extracellular space by astrocytes. In Huntington's disease GLU is bound

to the N-methyl-D-aspartate (NMDA) receptor resulting in an influx of calcium ions and subsequent cell death. This cascade of events with neuronal death most likely occurs in cerebrovascular accidents (e.g., stroke).

3. **Clinical signs** include choreiform movements, hypotonia, and progressive dementia.

D. **Other choreiform dyskinesias**

1. **Sydenham's chorea (St. Vitus' dance)** is the most common cause of chorea overall. It occurs primarily in girls, typically after a bout of rheumatic fever.

2. **Chorea gravidarum** usually occurs during the second trimester of pregnancy. Many patients have a history of Sydenham's chorea.

E. **Hemiballism** is a **movement disorder** that usually results from a vascular lesion of the subthalamic nucleus. Clinical signs include violent contralateral **flinging (ballistic) movements of one or both extremities.**

F. **Hepatolenticular degeneration (Wilson's disease)** is an **autosomal recessive disorder** that is caused by a defect in the **metabolism of copper.** The gene locus is on chromosome 13.

1. **Clinical signs** include choreiform or athetotic movements, rigidity, and **wing-beating tremor.** Tremor is the most common neurologic sign.

2. **Lesions** are found in the **lentiform nucleus.** Copper deposition in the limbus of the cornea gives rise to the **corneal Kayser-Fleischer ring,** which is a pathognomonic sign. Deposition of copper in the liver leads to multilobar cirrhosis.

3. **Psychiatric symptoms** include psychosis, personality disorders, and dementia.

4. The **diagnosis** is based on low serum ceruloplasmin, elevated urinary excretion of copper, and increased copper concentration in a liver biopsy specimen.

5. **Treatment** includes **penicillamine, a chelator.**

G. **Tardive dyskinesia** is a syndrome of **repetitive choreic movement** that **affects the face and trunk.** It results from treatment with phenothiazines, butyrophenones, or metoclopramide.

22

Neurotransmitters

I. IMPORTANT TRANSMITTERS AND THEIR PATHWAYS

A. Acetylcholine is the major transmitter of the peripheral nervous system, neuromuscular junction, parasympathetic nervous system, preganglionic sympathetic fibers, and postganglionic sympathetic fibers that innervate **sweat glands** and **some blood vessels** in the skeletal muscles (Figure 22-1). Acetylcholine is found in the neurons of the somatic and visceral motor nuclei in the brain stem and spinal cord. It is also found in the **basal nucleus of Meynert,** which degenerates in **Alzheimer's disease.**

B. Catecholamines. Figure 22-2 shows the biosynthetic pathway for catecholamines. Epinephrine, although a catecholamine, plays an insignificant role as a central nervous system neurotransmitter. In the body, epinephrine is found primarily in the adrenal medulla. In the central nervous system, it is restricted to small neuronal clusters in the brain stem (medulla).

1. Dopamine (Figure 22-3) is depleted in patients with Parkinson's disease and increased in patients with schizophrenia. Dopamine is found in the arcuate nucleus of the hypothalamus. It is the **prolactin-inhibiting factor.** Its two major receptors are D_1 and D_2.

Acetylcholine (ACh)

Figure 22-1. Distribution of acetylcholine-containing neurons and their axonal projections. The basal nucleus of Meynert projects to the entire cortex. This nucleus degenerates in patients with Alzheimer's disease. Striatal acetylcholine local circuit neurons degenerate in patients with Huntington's disease.

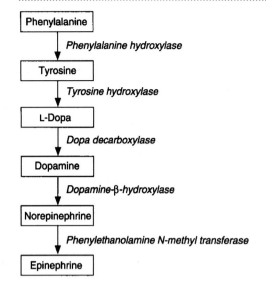

Figure 22-2. Synthesis of catecholamines from phenylalanine. Epinephrine, which is derived from norepinephrine, is found primarily in the adrenal medulla.

    a. D_1 receptors are postsynaptic. They activate adenylate cyclase and are excitatory.

    b. D_2 receptors are both postsynaptic and presynaptic. They inhibit adenylate cyclase and are inhibitory. Antipsychotic drugs block D_2 receptors.

  2. Norepinephrine (Figure 22-4) is the transmitter of most postganglionic sympathetic neurons. Antidepressant drugs enhance its transmission.

    a. Norepinephrine plays a role in **anxiety** states. **Panic attacks** are believed to result from paroxysmal discharges from the **locus ceruleus,** where norepinephrinergic neurons are found in the highest concentration. Most postsynaptic receptors of the locus ceruleus pathway are β_1 or β_2 receptors that activate adenylate cyclase and are excitatory.

Dopamine

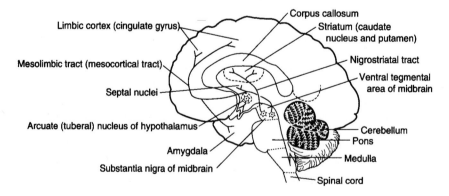

Figure 22-3. Distribution of dopamine-containing neurons and their projections. Two major ascending dopamine pathways arise in the midbrain: the nigrostriatal tract from the substantia nigra and the mesolimbic tract from the ventral tegmental area. In patients with Parkinson's disease, loss of dopaminergic neurons occurs in the substantia nigra and the ventral tegmental area. Dopaminergic neurons from the arcuate nucleus of the hypothalamus project to the portal vessels of the infundibulum. Dopaminergic neurons inhibit prolactin.

Norepinephrine (NE)

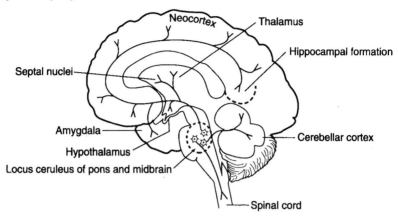

Figure 22-4. Distribution of norepinephrine-containing neurons and their projections. The locus ceruleus (located in the pons and midbrain) is the chief source of noradrenergic fibers. The locus ceruleus projects to all parts of the central nervous system.

  b. The **catecholamine hypothesis of mood disorders** states that reduced norepinephrine activity is related to depression, and that increased norepinephrine activity is related to mania.

C. Serotonin [5-hydroxytryptamine (5-HT)] is an indolamine (Figure 22-5). Serotonin-containing neurons are found only in the **raphe nuclei** of the brain stem.

  1. The **permissive serotonin hypothesis** states that when 5-HT activity is reduced, decreased levels of catecholamines cause depression and insomnia. In addition, when 5-HT activity is increased, elevated levels of catecholamines cause mania. Dysfunction of 5-HT may underlie obsessive-compulsive disorder.

  2. Certain **antidepressants** increase 5-HT availability by reducing its reuptake. 5-HT agonists that bind $5\text{-}HT_{1A}$ and those that block $5\text{-}HT_2$ have antidepressant properties. Fluoxetine is a selective serotonin reuptake inhibitor (SSRI).

D. Opioid peptides (endogenous opiates) induce responses similar to those of heroin and morphine.

  1. Endorphins include β-endorphin, which is the major endorphin found in the brain. It is one of the most powerful analgesics known (48 times more potent than morphine). Endorphins are found exclusively in the hypothalamus.

  2. Enkephalins are the most widely distributed and abundant opiate peptides. They are found in the highest concentration in the globus pallidus. Enkephalins coexist with dopamine, γ-aminobutyric acid (GABA), norepinephrine, and acetylcholine. They are colocalized in GABA-ergic pallidal neurons, and they play a role in pain suppression.

  3. Dynorphins follow the distribution map for enkephalins.

E. Nonopioid neuropeptides

  1. Substance P plays a role in **pain transmission.** It is most highly concentrated in the substantia nigra. It is also found in the dorsal root ganglion cells and substantia gelatinosa. It is colocalized with GABA in the striatonigral tract and plays a role in **movement disorders.** Substance P levels are **reduced** in patients with **Huntington's disease.**

Serotonin (5-HT)

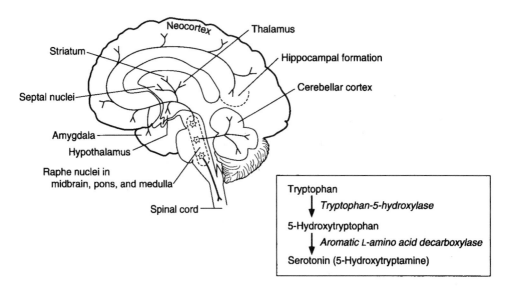

Figure 22-5.   Distribution of 5-hydroxytryptamine (serotonin)-containing neurons and their projections. Serotonin-containing neurons are found in the nuclei of the raphe. They project widely to the forebrain, cerebellum, and spinal cord. The *inset* shows the synthetic pathway of serotonin.

2. **Somatostatin (somatotropin-release inhibiting factor).** Somatostatinergic neurons from the anterior hypothalamus project their axons to the median eminence, where somatostatin enters the hypophyseal portal system and **regulates the release of growth hormone** and **thyroid-stimulating hormone.** The concentration of somatostatin in the neocortex and hippocampus is significantly **reduced** in patients with **Alzheimer's disease.** Striatal somatostatin levels are **increased** in patients with **Huntington's disease.**

F. **Amino acid transmitters**

1. **Inhibitory amino acid transmitters**

   a. **GABA** (Figure 22-6) is the major inhibitory neurotransmitter of the brain. Purkinje, stellate, basket, and Golgi cells of the cerebellar cortex are GABA-ergic.

      (1) **GABA-ergic striatal neurons** project to the globulus pallidus and substantia nigra.

      (2) **GABA-ergic pallidal neurons** project to the thalamus.

      (3) **GABA-ergic nigral neurons** project to the thalamus.

      (4) **GABA receptors** (GABA-A and GABA-B) are intimately associated with benzodiazepine-binding sites. Benzodiazepines enhance GABA activity.

         (a) **GABA-A receptors** open chloride channels.

         (b) **GABA-B receptors** are found on the terminals of neurons that use another transmitter (i.e., norepinephrine, dopamine, serotonin). Activation of GABA-B receptors decreases the release of the other transmitter.

   b. **Glycine** is the major inhibitory neurotransmitter of the spinal cord. It is used by the Renshaw cells of the spinal cord.

γ-Aminobutyric acid (GABA)

Figure 22-6. Distribution of γ-aminobutyric acid (GABA)-containing neurons and their projections. GABA-ergic neurons are the major inhibitory cells of the central nervous system. GABA local circuit neurons are found in the neocortex, hippocampal formation, and cerebellar cortex (Purkinje cells). Striatal GABA-ergic neurons project to the thalamus and subthalamic nucleus (not shown).

2. **Excitatory amino acid transmitters**

   a. **Glutamate** (Figure 22-7) is the **major excitatory transmitter of the brain.** Neocortical glutamatergic neurons project to the striatum, subthalamic nucleus, and thalamus.

      (1) Glutamate is the transmitter of the cerebellar granule cells.

      (2) Glutamate is also the transmitter of nonnociceptive, large, primary afferent fibers that enter the spinal cord and brain stem.

      (3) Glutamate is the transmitter of the corticobulbar and corticospinal tracts.

Glutamate

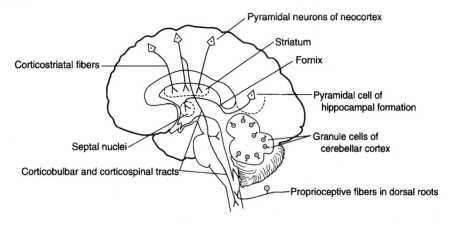

Figure 22-7. Distribution of glutamate-containing neurons and their projections. Glutamate is the major excitatory transmitter of the central nervous system. Cortical glutamatergic neurons project to the striatum. Hippocampal and subicular glutamatergic neurons project through the fornix to the septal area and hypothalamus. The granule cells of the cerebellum are glutamatergic.

  b. Aspartate, a major excitatory transmitter of the brain, is the transmitter of the climbing fibers of the cerebellum. Neurons of climbing fibers are found in the inferior olivary nucleus.

  c. Behavioral correlation. Glutamate, through its **N**-methyl-D-aspartate **(NMDA) receptors,** plays a role in **long-term potentiation** (a memory process) of hippocampal neurons. Glutamate plays a role in **kindling** and subsequent **seizure activity.** Under certain conditions, glutamate and its analogs are **neurotoxic.**

  d. Glutamate excitotoxicity. GLU is released in the striatum and binds to its receptors on striatal neurons resulting in an action potential. GLU is removed from the extracellular space by astrocytes. In Huntington's disease GLU is bound to the N-methyl-D-aspartate (NMDA) receptor resulting in an influx of calcium ions and subsequent cell death. This cascade of events with neuronal death most likely occurs in cerebrovascular accidents (stroke).

 3. Nitric oxide is a recently discovered gaseous neurotransmitter that is produced when nitric oxide-synthase converts arginine to citrulline.

  a. It is located in the olfactory system, striatum, neocortex, hippocampal formation, supraoptic nucleus of the hypothalamus, and cerebellum.

  b. Nitric oxide is responsible for smooth muscle relaxation of the corpus cavernosum and thus penile erection. It is also believed to play a role in memory formation because of its long-term potentiation in the hippocampal formation. In addition, nitric oxide functions as a nitrovasodilator in the cardiovascular system.

II. FUNCTIONAL AND CLINICAL CONSIDERATIONS

 A. Parkinson's disease results from degeneration of the dopaminergic neurons that are found in the pars compacta of the substantia nigra. It causes a reduction of dopamine in the striatum and substantia nigra (see Chapter 21 III A).

 B. Huntington's disease (chorea) results from a loss of acetylcholine- and GABA-containing neurons in the striatum (caudatoputamen). The effect is a loss of GABA in the striatum and substantia nigra (see Chapter 21 III C).

 C. Alzheimer's disease results from the degeneration of cortical neurons and cholinergic neurons in the **basal nucleus of Meynert.** It is associated with a 60% to 90% loss of choline acetyltransferase in the cerebral cortex. Histologically, **Alzheimer's disease** is characterized by the presence of **neurofibrillary tangles, senile (neuritic) plaques, amyloid substance, granulovacuolar degeneration, and Hirano bodies.**

 D. Myasthenia gravis results from autoantibodies against the nicotinic acetylcholine receptor on skeletal muscle. These antibodies block the postganglionic acetylcholine binding site. Thymic cells augment B-cell production of autoantibodies. The cardinal manifestation is fatigable weakness of the skeletal muscle. The extraocular muscles, including the levator palpebrae, are usually involved. Edrophonium or neostigmine injection is used for diagnosis.

 E. Lambert-Eaton myasthenic syndrome is caused by a presynaptic defect of acetylcholine release. It causes weakness in the limb muscles, but not the bulbar muscles. Fifty percent of cases are associated with neoplasms (i.e., lung, breast, prostate). In these patients, muscle strength improves with use. In contrast, in patients with myasthenia gravis, muscle use results in muscle fatigue, and autonomic dysfunction includes dry mouth, constipation, impotence, and urinary incontinence.

23
Cerebral Cortex

I. INTRODUCTION. The cerebral cortex, the thin, gray covering of both hemispheres of the brain, has two types: the neocortex (90%) and the allocortex (10%). Motor cortex is the thickest (4.5 mm); visual cortex is the thinest (1.5 mm).

II. THE SIX-LAYERED NEOCORTEX. Layers II and IV of the neocortex are mainly afferent (i.e., receiving). Layers V and VI are mainly efferent (i.e., sending) [Figure 23-1].

Figure 23-1. Neurocortical circuits. G = granule cell; H = horizontal cell; M = Martinotti cell; P = pyramidal cell; S = stellate cell. Loops show synaptic junctions. (Reprinted with permission from Parent A: *Carpenter's Human Neuroanatomy*, 9th ed. Baltimore, Williams & Wilkins, 1996, p. 868.)

A. Layer I is the **molecular** layer.

B. Layer II is the **external granular** layer.

C. Layer III is the **external pyramidal** layer. It gives rise to association and commissural fibers and is the major source of corticocortical fibers.

D. Layer IV is the **internal granular** layer. It receives thalamocortical fibers from the thalamic nuclei of the ventral tier (i.e., ventral posterolateral and ventral posteromedial). In the visual cortex (Brodmann's area 17), layer IV receives input from the lateral geniculate body.

E. Layer V is the **internal pyramidal** layer. It gives rise to corticobulbar, corticospinal, and corticostriatal fibers. It contains the giant pyramidal cells of Betz, which are found only in the motor cortex (Brodmann's area 4).

F. Layer VI is the **multiform** layer. It is the **major source of corticothalamic fibers.** It gives rise to projection, commissural, and association fibers.

III. FUNCTIONAL AREAS (Figure 23-2)

A. Frontal lobe

   1. The **motor cortex** (Brodmann's area 4) and **premotor cortex** (Brodmann's area 6) are somatotopically organized (Figure 23-3). Destruction of these areas of the frontal lobe causes contralateral spastic paresis. Contralateral pronator drift is associated with frontal lobe lesions of the corticospinal tract.

   2. **Frontal eye field** (Brodmann's area 8). Destruction causes deviation of the eyes to the ipsilateral side.

   3. **Broca's speech area** (Brodmann's areas 44 and 45) is located in the posterior part of the inferior frontal gyrus in the dominant hemisphere (Figure 23-4). Destruction results in expressive, nonfluent aphasia (Broca's aphasia). The patient understands both written and spoken language but cannot articulate speech or write normally. Broca's aphasia is usually associated with contralateral facial and arm weakness because of the involvement of the motor strip.

   4. **Prefrontal cortex** (Brodmann's areas 9–12 and 46–47). Destruction of the anterior two-thirds of the frontal lobe convexity results in deficits in concentration, orientation, abstracting ability, judgment, and problem-solving ability. Other frontal lobe deficits include loss of initiative, inappropriate behavior, release of sucking and grasping reflexes, gait apraxia, and sphincteric incontinence. Destruction of the orbital (frontal) lobe results in inappropriate social behavior (e.g., use of obscene language, urinating in public). Perseveration is associated with frontal lobe lesions.

B. Parietal lobe

   1. The **sensory cortex** (Brodmann's areas 3, 1, and 2) is somatotopically organized (see Figure 23-2). Destruction results in contralateral hemihypesthesia and astereognosis.

   2. The **superior parietal lobule** (Brodmann's areas 5 and 7). Destruction results in contralateral astereognosis and sensory neglect.

   3. The **inferior parietal lobule** of the **dominant hemisphere.** Damage results in Gerstmann's syndrome, which includes the following deficits:

     a. **Right and left confusion**

     b. **Finger agnosia**

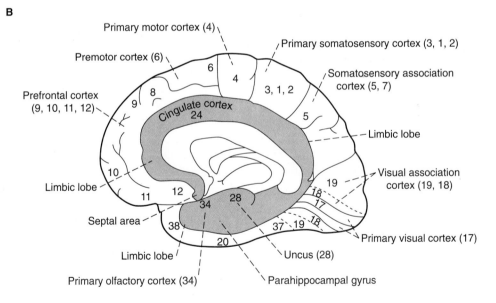

Figure 23-2. Some motor and sensory areas of the cerebral cortex. (A) Lateral convex surface of the hemisphere. (B) Medial surface of the hemisphere. The numbers refer to the Brodmann brain map (Brodmann's areas).

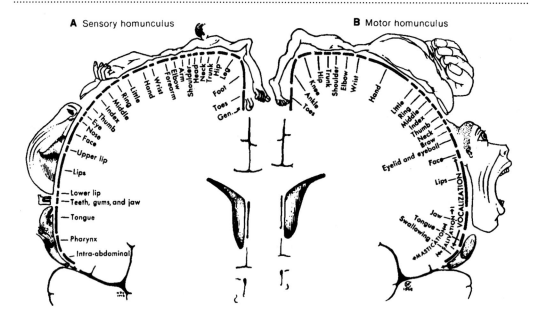

Figure 23-3.   The sensory and motor homunculi. (A) Sensory representation in the postcentral gyrus. (B) Motor representation in the precentral gyrus. (Reprinted with permission from Penfield W, Rasmussen T: *The Cerebral Cortex of Man*. New York, Hafner, 1968, pp. 44, 57.)

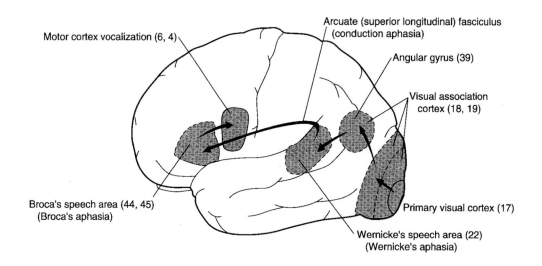

Figure 23-4.   Cortical areas of the dominant hemisphere that play an important role in language production. The visual image of a word is projected from the visual cortex (Brodmann's area 17) to the visual association cortices (Brodmann's areas 18 and 19) and then to the angular gyrus (Brodmann's area 39). Further processing occurs in Wernicke's speech area (Brodmann's area 22), where the auditory form of the word is recalled. Through the arcuate fasciculus, this information reaches Broca's speech area (Brodmann's areas 44 and 45), where motor speech programs control the vocalization mechanisms of the precentral gyrus. Lesions of Broca's speech area, Wernicke's speech area, or the arcuate fasciculus result in dysphasia. (Reprinted with permission from Fix JD: *BRS Neuroanatomy*, 3rd ed. Baltimore, Lippincott Williams & Wilkins, 2003, p. 377.)

   c. Dysgraphia and dyslexia

   d. Dyscalculia

   e. Contralateral hemianopia or lower quadrantanopia

4. The **inferior parietal lobule** of the **nondominant hemisphere.** Destruction results in the following deficits:

   a. Topographic memory loss

   b. Anosognosia

   c. Construction apraxia (Figure 23-5)

   d. Dressing apraxia

   e. Contralateral sensory neglect

   f. Contralateral hemianopia or lower quadrantanopia

C. Temporal lobe

1. The **primary auditory cortex** (Brodmann's areas 41 and 42). Unilateral destruction results in slight loss of hearing. Bilateral loss results in cortical deafness.

2. **Wernicke's speech area** in the **dominant hemisphere** is found in the posterior part of the superior temporal gyrus (Brodmann's area 22). Destruction results in receptive, fluent aphasia (Wernicke's aphasia), in which the patient cannot understand any form of language. Speech is spontaneous, fluent, and rapid, but makes little sense.

3. **Meyer's loop** (see Chapter 17 II F 2) consists of the visual radiations that project to the inferior bank of the calcarine sulcus. Interruption causes contralateral upper quadrantanopia ("pie in the sky").

4. **Olfactory bulb, tract,** and **primary cortex** (Brodmann's area 34). Destruction results in ipsilateral anosmia. An irritative lesion (psychomotor epilepsy) of the uncus results in olfactory and gustatory hallucinations.

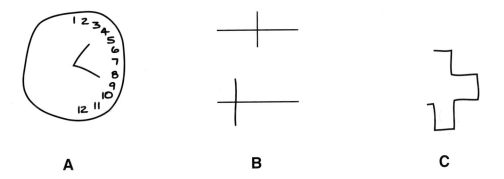

A   **B**   **C**

Figure 23-5.   Testing for construction apraxia. (A) The patient was asked to copy the face of a clock. (B) The patient was asked to bisect a horizontal line. (C) The patient was asked to copy a cross. These drawings show contralateral neglect. The responsible lesion is found in the nondominant (right) parietal lobe. A left hemianopia, by itself, does not result in contralateral neglect.

    a. **Olfactory groove meningiomas** compress the olfactory tract and bulb resulting in anosmia. See Foster Kennedy syndrome Chapter 13 I C.

    b. **Esthesioneuroblastomas** (olfactory neuroblastomas) arise from bipolar sensory cells of the olfactory mucosa; they can extend through the cribriform plate into the anterior cranial fossa. Presenting symptoms are similar to Foster Kennedy syndrome.

  5. **Hippocampal cortex (archicortex).** Bilateral lesions result in the inability to consolidate short-term memory into long-term memory. Earlier memories are retrievable.

  6. The **anterior temporal lobe,** including the **amygdaloid nucleus.** Bilateral damage results in **Kläver-Bucy** syndrome, which consists of **psychic blindness** (visual agnosia), **hyperphagia,** docility, and **hypersexuality.**

  7. **Inferomedial occipitotemporal cortex.** Bilateral lesions result in the inability to recognize once-familiar faces (prosopagnosia).

D. **Occipital lobe.** Bilateral lesions cause cortical blindness. Unilateral lesions cause contralateral hemianopia or quadrantanopia.

IV. **FOCAL DESTRUCTIVE HEMISPHERIC LESIONS AND SYMPTOMS.** Figure 23-6A shows the symptoms of lesions in the dominant hemisphere. Figure 23-6B shows the symptoms of lesions in the nondominant hemisphere.

V. **CEREBRAL DOMINANCE** is determined by the **Wada test.** Sodium amobarbital (Amytal) is injected into the carotid artery. If the patient becomes aphasic, the anesthetic was administered to the dominant hemisphere.

A. The **dominant hemisphere** is usually the left hemisphere. It is responsible for **propositional language** (grammar, syntax, and semantics), speech, and calculation.

B. The **nondominant hemisphere** is usually the right hemisphere. It is responsible for three-dimensional, or spatial, perception and nonverbal ideation. It also allows superior recognition of faces.

VI. **SPLIT-BRAIN SYNDROME** (Figure 23-7) is a disconnection syndrome that results from **transection** of the **corpus callosum.**

A. The **dominant hemisphere** is better at vocal naming.

B. The **nondominant, mute hemisphere** is better at pointing to a stimulus. A person cannot name objects that are presented to the nondominant visual cortex. A blindfolded person cannot name objects that are presented to the nondominant sensory cortex through touch.

C. Test (Figure 23-8). A subject views a composite picture of two half-faces (i.e., a chimeric, or hybrid, figure). The right side shows a man; the left side shows a woman. The picture is removed, and the subject is asked to describe what he saw. He may respond that he saw a man, but when asked to point to what he saw, he points to the woman.

D. In a patient who has **alexia** in the left visual field, the verbal symbols seen in the right visual cortex have no access to the language centers of the left hemisphere.

A

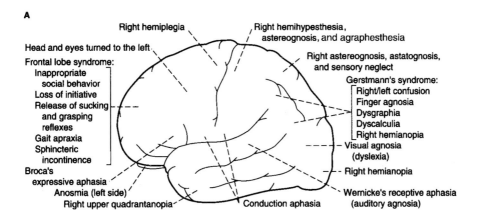

Right hemiplegia

Head and eyes turned to the left

Frontal lobe syndrome:
  Inappropriate
    social behavior
  Loss of initiative
  Release of sucking
    and grasping
    reflexes
  Gait apraxia
  Sphincteric
    incontinence

Broca's
  expressive aphasia
    Anosmia (left side)
      Right upper quadrantanopia

Right hemihypesthesia,
  astereognosis, and agraphesthesia

Right astereognosis, astatognosis,
  and sensory neglect

Gerstmann's syndrome:
  Right/left confusion
  Finger agnosia
  Dysgraphia
  Dyscalculia
  Right hemianopia

Visual agnosia
  (dyslexia)

Right hemianopia

Wernicke's receptive aphasia
  (auditory agnosia)

Conduction aphasia

B

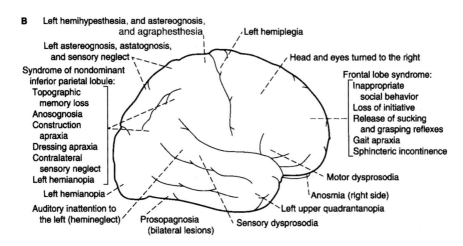

Left hemihypesthesia, and astereognosis,
  and agraphesthesia

Left astereognosis, astatognosis,
  and sensory neglect

Syndrome of nondominant
  inferior parietal lobule:
  Topographic
    memory loss
  Anosognosia
  Construction
    apraxia
  Dressing apraxia
  Contralateral
    sensory neglect
  Left hemianopia

Left hemianopia

Auditory inattention to
  the left (hemineglect)

Prosopagnosia
  (bilateral lesions)

Sensory dysprosodia

Left hemiplegia

Head and eyes turned to the right

Frontal lobe syndrome:
  Inappropriate
    social behavior
  Loss of initiative
  Release of sucking
    and grasping reflexes
  Gait apraxia
  Sphincteric incontinence

Motor dysprosodia

Anosmia (right side)

Left upper quadrantanopia

C

Contralateral spastic paresis in leg area

Incontinence

Contralateral hypesthesia in leg area

Contralateral sensory neglect

Inappropriate
  social behavior

Uncinate fits,
  with olfactory hallucinations

Klüver-Bucy
  syndrome

Contralateral lower
  quadrantanopia

Contralateral upper
  quadrantanopia

Defective memory
  consolidation (usually bilateral lesions)

Figure 23-6.   Focal destructive hemispheric lesions and the resulting symptoms. (A) Lateral convex surface of the dominant left hemisphere. (B) Lateral convex surface of the nondominant right hemisphere. (C) Medial surface of the nondominant hemisphere.

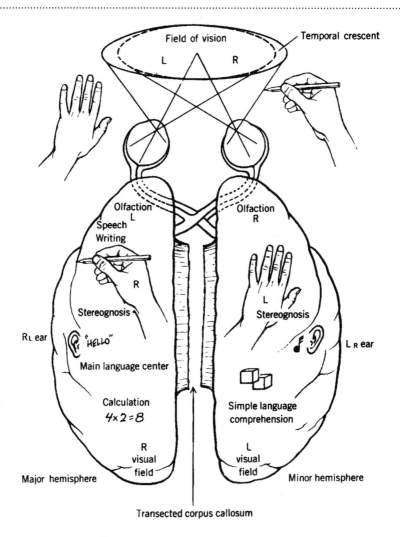

Figure 23-7. Functions of the split brain after transection of the corpus callosum. Tactile and visual perception is projected to the contralateral hemisphere, olfaction is perceived on the same side, and audition is perceived predominantly in the opposite hemisphere. The left (L) hemisphere is dominant for language. The right (R) hemisphere is dominant for spatial construction and nonverbal ideation. (Reprinted with permission from Noback CR, Demarest RJ: *The Human Nervous System*. Malvern, PA, Lea & Febiger, 1991, p. 416.)

VII. OTHER LESIONS OF THE CORPUS CALLOSUM

   A. **Anterior corpus callosum lesion** may result in akinetic mutism or tactile anomia.

   B. **Posterior corpus callosum (splenium) lesion** may result in alexia without agraphia.

   C. **Callosotomy** has been successfully used to treat "drop attacks" (colloid cyst of third ventricle).

VIII. BRAIN AND SPINAL CORD TUMORS (see Chapter 5)

Figure 23-8. Chimeric (hybrid) figure of a face used to examine the hemispheric function of commissurotomized patients. The patient is instructed to fixate on the dot and is asked to describe what he sees. If he says that he sees the face of a man, then the left hemisphere predominates in vocal tasks. If he is asked to point to the face and he points to the woman, then the right hemisphere predominates in pointing tasks.

24

Apraxia, Aphasia, and Dysprosody

I. APRAXIA is the inability to perform motor activities in the presence of intact motor and sensory systems and normal comprehension.

A. Ideomotor apraxia (Idiokenetic apraxia)

1. Loss of the ability to perform intransitive or imaginary gestures; the inability to perform complicated motor tasks (e.g., saluting, blowing a kiss or making the "V" for victory sign)

2. The lesion is in Wernicke's area

3. Bucco-facial or facial-oral apraxia is a type of idiomotor apraxia; facial apraxia is the most common type of apraxia

B. Ideational apraxia (Ideatory apraxia)

1. The inability to demonstrate the use of real objects (e.g., ask the patient to smoke a pipe (a multistep complex sequence)

2. A misuse of objects due to a disturbance of identification (agnosia)

3. The lesion is in Wernicke's area

C. Construction apraxia is the inability to draw or construct a geometric figure (e.g., the face of a clock). If the patient draws only the right half of the clock, this condition is called hemineglect, and the lesion is located in the right inferior parietal lobule (see Figure 23-4).

D. Gait apraxia is the inability to use the lower limbs properly. The patient has difficulty in lifting his feet from the floor, a frontal lobe sign seen with **normal pressure hydrocephalus (gait apraxia, dementia, incontinence).**

II. APHASIA is impaired or absent communication by speech, writing, or signs (i.e., loss of the capacity for spoken language). The lesions are located in the dominant hemisphere. Associate the following symptoms and lesion sites with the appropriate aphasia (Figure 24-1).

A. Broca's (motor) aphasia

1. Lesion in frontal lobe, in the inferior frontal gyrus (Brodmann 44, 45)

2. Good comprehension

3. Effortful speech

4. Dysarthric speech

Appendix: Table of Cranial Nerves

Cranial Nerve	Type	Origin	Function	Course
I—Olfactory	SVA	Bipolar olfactory olfactory epithelium in roof of nasal cavity)	Smell (olfaction)	Central axons project to the olfactory bulb via the cribriform plate of the ethmoid bone.
II—Optic	SSA	Retinal ganglion cells	Vision	Central axons converge at the optic disk and form the optic nerve, which enters the skull via the optic canal. Optic nerve axons terminate in the lateral geniculate bodies.
III—Oculomotor				
Parasympathetic	GVE	Edinger-Westphal nucleus (rostral midbrain)	Sphincter muscle of iris; ciliary muscle	Axons exit the midbrain in the interpeduncular fossa, traverse the cavernous sinus, and enter
Motor	GSE	Oculomotor nucleus (rostral midbrain)	Superior, inferior, and medial recti muscles; inferior oblique muscle; levator palpebrae muscle	the orbit via the superior orbital fissure.
IV—Trochlear	GSE	Trochlear nucleus (caudal midbrain)	Superior oblique muscle	Axons decussate in superior medullary velum, exit dorsally inferior to the inferior colliculi, encircle the midbrain, traverse the cavernous sinus, and enter the orbit via the superior orbital fissure.
V—Trigeminal				
Motor	SVE	Motor nucleus CN V (mid pons)	Muscles of mastication and tensor tympani muscle	Ophthalmic nerve exits via the superior orbital fissure; maxillary nerve exits via the foramen rotundum; mandibular
Sensory	GSA	Trigeminal ganglion and mesencephalic nucleus CN V (rostral pons and midbrain)	Tactile, pain, and thermal sensation from the face; the oral and nasal cavities; and the supratentorial dura	nerve exits via the foramen ovale; ophthalmic and maxillary nerves traverse the cavernous sinus; GSA fibers enter the spinal trigeminal tract of CN V.
VI—Abducent	GSE	Abducent nucleus (caudal pons)	Lateral rectus muscle	Axons exit the pons from the inferior pontine sulcus, traverse the cavernous sinus, and enter the orbit via the superior orbital fissure.

(continued)

Appendix: (continued)

Cranial Nerve	Type	Origin	Function	Course
VII—Facial				Axons exit the pons in the cerebellar pontine angle and enter the internal auditory meatus; motor fibers traverse the facial canal of the temporal bone and exit via the stylomastoid foramen; taste fibers traverse the chorda tympani and lingual nerve; GSA fibers enter the spinal trigeminal tract of CN V; SVA fibers enter the tract.
Parasympathetic	GVE	Superior salivatory nucleus (caudal pons)	Lacrimal gland (via sphenopalatine ganglion); submandibular and sublingual glands (via submandibular ganglion)	
Motor	SVE	Facial nucleus (caudal pons)	Muscles of facial expression; stapedius muscle	
Sensory	GSA	Geniculate ganglion (temporal bone)	Tactile sensation to skin of ear	
Sensory	SVA	Geniculate ganglion	Taste sensation from the anterior two-thirds of tongue (via chorda tympani)	
VIII—Vestibulocochlear	SSA			Vestibular and cochlear nerves join in the internal auditory meatus and enter the brain stem in the cerebellopontine angle; vestibular nerve projects to the vestibular nuclei and the flocculonodular lobe of the cerebellum; cochlear nerve projects to the cochlear nuclei
Vestibular nerve		Vestibular ganglion (internal auditory meatus)	Equilibrium (innervates hair cells of semicircular ducts, saccule, and utricle)	
Cochlear nerve		Spiral ganglion (modiolus of temporal bone)	Hearing (innervates hair cells of the organ of Corti)	
IX—Glossopharyngeal				Axons exit (motor) and enter (sensory) medulla from the postolivary sulcus; axons exit and enter the skull via jugular foramen; GSA fibers enter the spinal trigeminal-tract of CN V; GVA and SVA fibers enter the solitary tract.
Parasympathetic	GVE	Inferior salivatory nucleus (rostral medulla)	Parotid gland (via the otic ganglion)	
Motor	SVE	Nucleus ambiguus (rostral medulla)	Stylopharyngeus muscle	
Sensory	GSA	Superior ganglion (jugular foramen)	Tactile sensation to external ear	
Sensory	GVA	Inferior (petrosal) ganglion (in jugular foramen)	Tactile sensation to posterior third of tongue, pharynx, middle ear, and auditory tube; input from carotid sinus and carotid body	
Sensory	SVA	Inferior (petrosal) ganglion (in jugular foramen)	Taste from posterior third of the tongue	

(continued)

Appendix: (continued)

Cranial Nerve	Type	Origin	Function	Course
X—Vagal				Axons exit (motor) and enter (sensory) medulla from the postolivary sulcus; axons exit and enter the skull via the jugular foramen; GSA fibers enter the spinal trigeminal tract of CN V; GVA and SVA fibers enter the solitary tract.
Parasympa-thetic	GVE	Dorsal nucleus of CN X (medulla)	Viscera of the thoracic and abdominal cavities to the left colic flexure [via terminal (mural) ganglia]	
Motor	SVE	Nucleus ambiguus (midmedulla)	Muscles of the larynx and pharynx	
Sensory	GSA	Superior ganglion (jugular foramen)	Tactile sensation to the external ear	
Sensory	GVA	Inferior (nodose) ganglion (in jugular foramen)	Mucous membranes of the pharynx, larynx, esophagus, trachea, and thoracic and abdominal viscera to the left colic flexure	
Sensory	SVA	Inferior (nodose) ganglion (in jugular foramen)	Taste from the epiglottis	
XI—Accessory	SVE			Axons from the cranial division exit the medulla from the postolivary sulcus and join the vagal nerve; axons from spinal division exit the spinal cord, ascend through the foramen magnum, and exit the skull via the jugular foramen.
Motor (cranial)		Nucleus ambiguus (medulla)	Intrinsic muscles of the larynx (except the cricothyroid muscle) via recurrent laryngeal nerve	
Motor (spinal)		Ventral horn neurons C1–C6	Sternocleidomastoid and trapezius muscles	
XII—Hypoglossal	GSE	Hypoglossal nucleus (medulla)	Intrinsic and extrinsic muscles of the tongue (except the palatoglossus muscle)	Axons exit from the preolivary sulcus of the medulla and exit the skull via the hypoglossal canal.

SVA = special visceral afferent; SSA = special somatic afferent; GVE = general visceral efferent; GSE = general somatic efferent; SVE = special visceral efferent; GSA = general somatic afferent; GVA = general visceral afferent; CN = cranial nerve.

Index

Italic page numbers designate figures; page numbers followed by "t" designate tables; (*see also*) refers to related topics or more detailed topic breakdowns. Topics having more than one subentry are listed under the noun (e.g., Body (bodies): carotid).